menopause guidebook

MW00815315

table of contents

MENOPAUSE BASICS

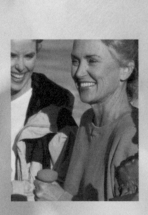

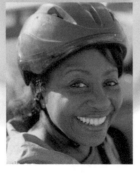

MENOPAUSE IS THE END OF

MENSTRUATION, USUALLY CONFIRMED

WHEN A WOMAN HAS NOT HAD

A MENSTRUAL PERIOD FOR

12 CONSECUTIVE MONTHS, IN THE

ABSENCE OF OTHER OBVIOUS CAUSES.

MENOPAUSE IS ASSOCIATED WITH

REDUCED FUNCTIONING OF THE

OVARIES AND THE RESULTING

VARIATION AND ULTIMATE DECLINE

IN A WOMAN'S LEVEL OF OVARIAN

HORMONES, INCLUDING ESTROGEN,

PROGESTERONE, AND ANDROGEN.

MENOPAUSE ALSO MARKS THE END

OF FERTILITY.

Menopause is a normal, natural event – not a disease. As a woman moves from her reproductive years through the menopause transition and beyond, physical changes occur. Most of these changes are normal, but others may suggest illness. Some changes are related to menopause, while others are more related to aging. It is often difficult to distinguish menopause-related changes from age-related changes, because conditions not related to menopause – such as obesity, diabetes, thyroid disorders, or hypertension – often develop during midlife.

Menopause eventually happens to all women, but it affects each woman uniquely. For some, the end of fertility brings a sense of freedom as concerns about birth control and menstrual periods cease. For others, menopause can contribute to serious health problems when hormone levels change and the physical effects of aging are coupled with the stresses of midlife. For most women, menopause is a passageway to a new part of life when they report feeling more confident, empowered, involved, and energized than in their younger years. One thing, however, is true for all women. Menopause signals an opportunity to enhance quality of life through improved health practices.

TIMING AND TERMINOLOGY

Defined below are several terms used when describing the menopause experience.

Natural Menopause

Natural menopause is a spontaneous, permanent ending of menstruation that is not caused by any medical intervention. In the Western world, most women experience natural menopause between the ages of 40 and 58, with the average at about age 51. Some women reach natural menopause as early as their 30s and a few in their 60s.

Women often experience menopause around the same age as their mothers and sisters, but contrary to previous opinion, there is no correlation between a woman's age at menopause and the time of her first period or whether she used oral contraceptives. There is limited evidence to associate being underweight with earlier menopause and being overweight with later menopause. Other than genetics, cigarette smoking is the only factor proven to affect age at menopause. Smokers, and even former smokers, can reach menopause one to two years earlier than nonsmokers.

Perimenopause

Perimenopause literally means "around menopause." It is what some call "being in menopause," but menopause is really only one day in a woman's life.

Perimenopause refers to the transition time that begins immediately prior to natural menopause when menstrual cycles become irregular. It can last up to six years or more, and it ends the first year after menopause. Perimenopausal changes are brought on by changes in ovarian hormone production and the hormones that regulate them. Irregular menstrual periods, hot flashes, vaginal dryness, difficulty sleeping, and mood swings are common, normal signs of perimenopause.

> *Menopause is a normal, natural event – not a disease.*

Induced Menopause

Induced menopause is an immediate menopause brought on by surgical removal of the ovaries or ovarian damage as a result of medical interventions such as cancer chemotherapy or pelvic radiation.

Induced menopause brought on by surgical removal of both ovaries is called surgical menopause. Menstrual bleeding stops, and the woman is no longer fertile. A hysterectomy removes the uterus, but if the ovaries are left in place and continue to produce hormones, it does not induce menopause,

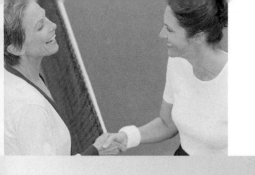

Menopause is a signal to start or to continue a good health program.

even though menstrual bleeding stops and the woman can no longer bear children. Even if the ovaries are left in place, a hysterectomy can bring on natural menopause a year or two earlier than expected. Hysterectomy in younger women can sometimes disturb the blood supply to the ovaries, causing hot flashes. Women who have had a hysterectomy will still go through perimenopause as their ovaries gradually secrete less estrogen. But without a uterus, a woman will no longer menstruate, and so she will not have the most reliable indicator of the beginning of perimenopause – irregular periods.

Premenopausal women who experience induced menopause do not go through perimenopause. Instead, they are faced with menopause and its implications without a period of gradual adjustment. Because of the abrupt loss of ovarian hormones, including estrogen, these women may have more intense menopause-related disturbances, such as hot flashes. Because they spend more years than most women without the protective effects of estrogen, they may also be at greater risk later in life for such health problems as the bone-thinning disease of osteoporosis and, possibly, heart disease.

The emotional impact of induced menopause may also be greater than with natural menopause. Women must often cope with the disease or condition that led to their need for medical intervention as well as the side effects of therapy. For example, pelvic radiation can cause hot flashes and severe vaginal dryness and irritation. Chemotherapy, depending on which drugs are used, may cause hair loss, nausea, fatigue, weight gain, and lack of energy, in addition to its effect on the ovaries.

Another important difference between natural and induced menopause is the need for treatment. Typically, women experiencing induced menopause have a greater need for treatment to control the acute symptoms and, potentially, to lower the risk of some diseases later in life. Very little is known about the long-term risk-reduction benefits of hormone use in younger women; all the studies are with post-menopausal women. There is also a concern about use of hormones for many years. Many times, hormones are not an option for medical reasons, and alternatives must be considered.

Sometimes a woman using certain drugs called GnRH analogues (sometimes used to treat endometriosis, severe PMS, and uterine fibroids) can experience a temporary cessation of menstrual periods. When therapy is discontinued, the ovaries usually resume normal production of estrogen and other hormones. Lifestyle-related issues, such as high levels of emotional stress and over-exercising, and excessive dieting, including eating disorders such as anorexia and bulimia, can also stop periods. Normal function usually resumes when more healthful habits are adopted.

Premature Menopause

Menopause, whether natural or induced, is called premature when it is reached before age 40. Premature menopause can be the result of genetics, autoimmune processes, or medical interventions, such as surgical removal of ovaries, chemotherapy, or pelvic radiation. Premature menopause places a woman at increased risk for osteoporosis and, possibly, heart disease over the rest of her life.

Because premature menopause means the end of natural childbearing, it can be a source of psychological distress. Many younger women grieve the loss of fertility and the children they will never have. Some women link fertility with their concept of femininity and sexual desirability, so addressing the psychological impact of premature menopause is as important as addressing the physical impact.

For women who still desire pregnancy, donor egg programs may be an option.

Premature menopause and premature ovarian failure (POF) share some of the same characteristics. However, POF is not always permanent and, thus, the terms should not be used interchangeably.

Postmenopause

Postmenopause refers to all the years beyond menopause – whether induced or natural.

CONFIRMING MENOPAUSE STATUS

Perimenopause is usually confirmed through a review of a woman's medical history and the changes she is experiencing (such as irregular periods and hot flashes) as well as by ruling out any other cause for these changes. In most cases, hormone tests aren't needed, since therapy, if required, is usually based on a woman's symptoms or concerns. If there is a question regarding hormone levels, tests may be used.

The most reliable test measures the blood level of the follicle-stimulating hormone (FSH), a hormone produced by the pituitary gland to stimulate the ovaries to secrete estrogen. As the aging ovaries' production of estrogen declines, the pituitary gland tries to stimulate greater estrogen production by releasing more FSH into the blood.

When a woman's FSH rises to a consistent blood level of 30 to 40 mIU/mL or higher, it is generally accepted that she has reached menopause. However, FSH levels can be misleading since estrogen production doesn't fall steadily day to day during perimenopause. Instead, estrogen levels fluctuate, with days or weeks of fairly high or fairly low levels of production. Therefore, more than one FSH measurement is needed to confirm menopause. It is important to note that if a woman is using certain hormonal contraceptives (such as birth control pills), an FSH test will not be valid.

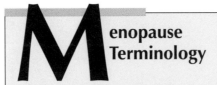

Menopause Terminology

Menopause is the end of menstruation, confirmed after 12 consecutive months without a period or when the ovaries are removed or damaged.

Perimenopause is the transitional time of up to six years or more immediately prior to natural menopause when changes begin, plus one year after menopause.

Induced menopause is the immediate menopause caused by a medical or surgical intervention that removes or damages both ovaries.

Premature menopause is menopause that occurs before age 40.

Postmenopause is all the years beyond menopause.

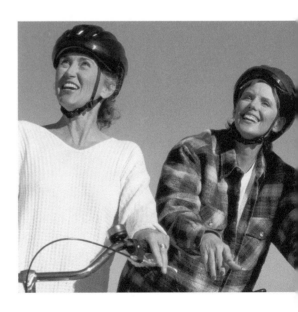

PERIMENOPAUSAL CHANGES

SOME TYPICAL PERIMENOPAUSAL CHANGES ARE REDUCED FERTILITY, IRREGULAR MENSTRUAL PERIODS, HOT FLASHES, URINARY AND GENITAL CHANGES, CHANGES IN SEXUAL FUNCTION, AND MOOD CHANGES. THEY ARE OCCASIONALLY CALLED SYMPTOMS EVEN THOUGH MENOPAUSE IS NOT A DISEASE AND THIS TERM IS USUALLY RESERVED TO DESCRIBE DISEASES.

Many changes during perimenopause are normal and natural. They usually start when a woman is in her 40s, sometimes even in her 30s. As a rule, most will not continue far beyond menopause, and will stop without treatment. Some changes are problematic and need treatment. All changes, however, signal the need for a medical evaluation because it cannot be assumed that hot flashes and other changes are caused by approaching menopause. Some changes can be signals of disease or can be caused by other ailments, such as a thyroid disorder. Therefore, it is advisable to report any changes to a healthcare provider.

A woman's response to the physical changes of the perimenopausal years, while not genetically determined, can often be predicted by her mother's response. Women whose mothers describe their menopause as terrible may become conditioned to have a similar experience. Hot flashes or other discomforts of menopause are very real, yet the level of distress that a woman experiences is partly based on her expectations.

For some women, menopause just means the end of menstrual periods. To others, it means uncertainty about what to expect and an unwelcome reminder that they are aging. But women who embrace the changes, rather than dreading them, are the ones who find menopause to be an event that brings about better relationships and greater personal fulfillment, and they are more likely to make lifestyle changes that will improve their health for the rest of their lives. Women today are living in an era when menopause is better understood than ever before, and they have the advantage of being able to talk openly about it.

REDUCED FERTILITY

Beginning late in their 30s, women's fertility typically begins to wane significantly, primarily due to aging eggs in the ovaries. While there are many fertility-enhancing techniques available for midlife women, they are expensive, have some risks, and are not always successful. At the same time, the risk of spontaneous miscarriage begins to rise, reaching about 50% by age 45. Also at this age, the risk of a genetic abnormality in a fetus is 1 in 40, and there is an increased chance of pregnancy complications, such as gestational diabetes, stillbirth, and the need for cesarean section.

BIRTH CONTROL AS MENOPAUSE APPROACHES

Information about birth control in a menopause booklet may seem surprising. But, despite a decline in fertility during perimenopause, women are not totally protected from an unplanned pregnancy until menopause is reached. If pregnancy is not desired, it is important to choose an effective, safe, and appropriate method of birth control, particularly in midlife when pregnancy can have an impact on health far beyond the reproductive years.

Birth Control Options

Midlife women have a wide range of effective birth control options. A healthcare provider can help determine the best birth control choice based on a woman's medical history, lifestyle, and sexual habits. It should be noted that only one method – condom use – provides protection from HIV and other sexually transmitted infections (STIs). Options include the following:

Sterilization methods include tubal ligation (for women) and vasectomy (for men). **Pros:** These methods are safe and have a very low failure rate of about 4 to 8 in 1,000. Tubal ligation (having tubes "tied") does not cause menopause. **Cons:** They are surgical procedures and have to be considered permanent.

Changes during perimenopause are normal and natural, but they do signal a need for a medical evaluation.

Barrier methods include the diaphragm, cervical cap, spermicides, and the male and female condom. **Pros:** These methods are highly effective if used during every act of vaginal sex, although spermicide alone is less effective. A condom is the only method proven effective as protection against both pregnancy and STIs when used during vaginal, oral, and anal sex. Condoms can be used in combination with other birth control methods, and they are available without a prescription. **Cons:** A few women and men are allergic to latex condoms or certain spermicides. These methods must be used during every act of sex, and condoms may break, leak, or spill when removed.

Oral contraceptives, sometimes called birth control pills, contain either one hormone (progestin) or two (progestin plus estrogen) for contraception. **Pros:** These prescription products provide effective contraception; after discontinuing use, there is a rapid return of fertility. Modern low-dose pills that combine estrogen and progestin are safe for healthy, nonsmoking, midlife women, and are highly effective when taken as directed. Noncontraceptive benefits include reduced risk of ovarian and endometrial cancer, fewer fibrocystic breast changes, and reduced rates of postmenopausal bone density loss. They may also help regulate periods and reduce hot flashes during perimenopause. Long-term use will not significantly increase cardiovascular risk in healthy nonsmokers. Most studies do not show a significant relationship between use of birth control pills and risk of breast cancer.

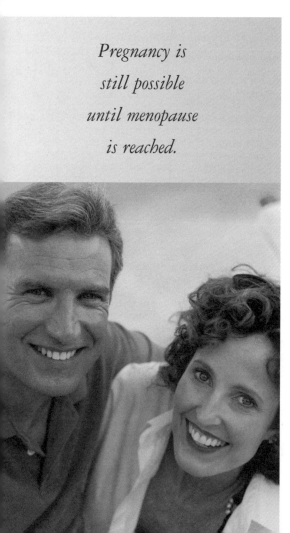

Pregnancy is still possible until menopause is reached.

Cons: Contraindications include history of blood clots or coronary artery disease, breast cancer, jaundice during previous birth control pill use, pregnancy or suspected pregnancy, uncontrolled hypertension, and cigarette smoking in women over age 35. Possible side effects include nausea, breast tenderness, new or worsening headaches, and spotting between periods. Using birth control pills can mask changes in a woman's period, and thereby mute her natural signal of approaching menopause. Birth control pills also invalidate the FSH test that is often used to confirm menopause. Because of the difficulty in knowing when menopause is reached, most clinicians advise women to stop birth control pills at age 51, the average age of menopause. Heart attack and stroke are rare but serious side effects, especially in smokers and with the use of older high-dose pills. The mini-pill, which contains only a progestin, may be better for women at risk for blood clots in the legs (phlebitis). However, the mini-pill is slightly less effective in preventing pregnancy than the combination pills and may not offer the same noncontraceptive health benefits.

Progestin injections. Two injectable birth control options are available: Depo-Provera and Lunelle. Both contain progestin for effectiveness, and both require a healthcare provider to give the injection into a large muscle (typically the buttocks). Lunelle also contains estrogen. **Pros:** A single injection of one of these products provides more than 99% contraceptive effectiveness for several weeks (up to one month for Lunelle and up to three months for Depo-Provera). Long-term use is associated with lower uterine cancer risk. After discontinuing use, fertility returns rapidly with Lunelle and within one year for Depo-Provera. **Cons:** Contraindications include pregnancy, vaginal bleeding of unknown cause, breast cancer, liver disease, and blood clotting disorders. Common side effects include weight gain, hair loss, and changes in menstrual cycle, especially during the first few months of use. Other possible effects are fatigue, headaches, nervousness, and dizziness. They also require regular visits to the healthcare provider for injections (monthly for Lunelle and every three months for Depo-Provera).

Intrauterine devices (IUDs) can be placed inside the uterus by a clinician. Different devices use different materials for effectiveness, such as copper or a progestogen. **Pros:** IUDs are highly effective for long-term pregnancy protection (up to five years for one progestogen device, 10 years for copper). Today's IUDs are much safer and more effective than older devices, and there is no evidence of increased risk of pelvic inflammatory disease or cancer. When removed, contraception is reversed and fertility rapidly restored. **Cons:** Contraindications include pregnancy or suspicion of pregnancy, history of pelvic inflammatory disease, not being in a mutually monogamous relationship, abnormality of the reproductive system (which includes an unresolved abnormal Pap test), abnormal genital bleeding, anemia, and infection of the fallopian tubes or ovaries. Possible side effects of cramping or spotting may occur initially after insertion. In addition, menstrual periods may be heavier and last longer while the IUD is in place, although one of the progestogen-containing IUDs has been found to reduce bleeding by up to 90%. The office procedure for insertion may be uncomfortable, and cramping or spotting may occur initially. The user must periodically check the string that remains outside the uterus in the vagina to ensure the IUD is in place. The string is sometimes felt by the partner. IUD use requires at least an annual exam by a clinician.

Progestin implant system. One implant system, Norplant, is available for birth control and consists of six match-sized, progestin-releasing capsules that are surgically implanted by a clinician under the skin of the inner, upper arm. **Pros:** The implants, which can be removed by the clinician at any time, offer 98% contraceptive effectiveness. When removed, fertility returns rapidly. **Cons:** Contraindications include pregnancy, history of blood clots, unexplained vaginal bleeding, breast cancer, or liver disease.

Side effects include headaches, nausea, weight change, acne, increased vaginal dryness, and irregular uterine bleeding, typically in the first 9 to 12 months after insertion. Some medications used for epilepsy may make the implants less effective. The system's costs include purchasing the product plus the office surgery to insert and remove the capsules. Implants must be removed after five years, and there is a possibility of permanent scarring at the insertion site.

Methods that use no drugs, devices, or surgery include natural family planning, such as rhythm or periodic abstinence. **Pros:** There is no cost, no need to take drugs or use devices, and no need for surgery. There are no contraindications or side effects. **Cons:** When using the rhythm method, it is especially difficult to predict unsafe days during perimenopause when periods are irregular.

Emergency Contraception

The use of "emergency contraception" can be effective if used within 72 hours of unexpected, unprotected sex or a condom accident. These "morning-after" pills should not be used as regular birth control.

CHANGES IN MENSTRUAL PERIODS

During the reproductive years, two of the hormones made by the ovaries – estrogen and progesterone – play important roles in the menstrual cycle. In preparation for a fertilized egg, estrogen causes the endometrium (lining of the uterus) to start to thicken. Progesterone then causes a ripening or secretion of nutrients.

If a fertilized egg is not received in the uterus, the ovaries stop making these hormones, and the uterine lining is shed as the menstrual period. Each woman has a pattern to her periods, which differs from woman to woman.

A few women simply stop menstruating one day and never have another period. Most women, however, go though a longer perimenopause and experience changes or irregularities in their menstrual periods. These irregularities are caused by secretion of erratic levels of ovarian hormones and decreased frequency of egg release (ovulation). Initially, the menstrual changes can be subtle. Usually a woman's cycle will get shorter, with periods occurring more often than every 28 days. Bleeding may last fewer or more days than previously, and blood flow may be heavier, lighter, or just spotting. Late in perimenopause, skipping periods becomes common. However, some women skip several cycles and then menstruate regularly again. Any menstrual pattern is possible – but each woman will know that, for her, a change has occurred.

A menstrual diary is helpful to determine what's normal or abnormal.

For most women, these changes are natural and normal during perimenopause, and no treatments are needed.

Normal vs Abnormal Menstrual Bleeding

Irregular periods are common and normal during perimenopause, but it should not be assumed that all changes in uterine bleeding are simply due to menopause. Other conditions may cause abnormal bleeding, so a healthcare provider should be consulted if any of the following conditions appear:

- Periods are very heavy or gushing, or accompanied by clots;

- Periods last more than seven days, or two or more days longer than usual;

- Intervals are shorter than 21 days from the start of one period to the start of the next;

- Spotting or uterine bleeding happens between menstrual periods;

- Bleeding from the vagina occurs after intercourse.

Possible causes of abnormal perimenopausal bleeding include the following:

Hormonal imbalance. Irregular or heavy bleeding can be caused by an imbalance in ovarian estrogen and progesterone production or by an imbalance of another hormone (such as when a woman has either high or low thyroid hormone levels).

Hormonal contraceptives. Use of products such as prescription contraceptive pills, implants, injections, and intrauterine devices can cause spotting or breakthrough bleeding, particularly in younger women. Spotting refers to a small amount of bleeding from the vagina that occurs at the monthly time for a period. Breakthrough bleeding occurs at a time other than the monthly time for a period.

Pregnancy. Until menopause is reached, pregnancy can occur and cause abnormal uterine bleeding as well as missed periods.

Fibroids. These noncancerous growths in or around the uterus are a very common cause of abnormal uterine bleeding. While some fibroid tumors produce no symptoms, others can produce dramatic changes in periods (such as prolonged and/or heavy bleeding), menstrual cramps, back pain, and difficulty with bowel movements or urination. While the cause of fibroids is unknown, their growth can be stimulated by estrogen surges that sometimes occur during perimenopause. Fibroids may shrink after menopause when the ovaries reduce production of estrogen. Occasionally, estrogen replacement therapy stimulates their growth once more.

Uterine lining (endometrium) abnormalities. Noncancerous growths, such as polyps, in the endometrium can result in abnormal uterine bleeding.

Cancer. In a very small percentage of cases, some types of cancer in the uterus, vagina, and cervix can cause abnormal bleeding from the uterus and/or vagina. Regular pelvic exams and Pap smears are particularly helpful in diagnosing these serious diseases early enough for effective treatment.

Other causes. Factors that interfere with blood clotting sometimes cause uterine bleeding. In addition, although bleeding passing from the vagina usually comes from the uterus, it is possible for the vagina or cervix to be the source of bleeding.

> *Do not assume that all changes in uterine bleeding are due to menopause-related hormone changes.*

Finding the Cause

There are several procedures a clinician can use to determine the cause of abnormal uterine bleeding, including the following:

Endometrial biopsy. This is a widely used procedure often performed in a clinician's office, and no anesthesia is needed. A small sample of the uterine lining is removed through the cervix (opening to the uterus from the vagina) then examined by a pathologist. Endometrial biopsy is often used to exclude cancer, and it can sometimes identify other reasons for bleeding.

Dilation and curettage (D&C). In this surgical procedure, the cervix is dilated and the uterine lining removed by scraping or by suction and scraping. Because it usually requires anesthesia, D&C has

been performed less frequently since the advent of the endometrial biopsy.

Hysteroscopy. In this procedure, a tiny telescope is inserted into the vagina and through the cervix to view the uterine lining directly. A biopsy can usually be done at the same time if there are any observed abnormalities.

Transvaginal ultrasound. This painless procedure uses sound-generated images, similar to the ultrasound images used during pregnancy. The images are obtained with a probe inserted into the vagina. Although it is less invasive than surgery, transvaginal ultrasound can sometimes miss small abnormalities.

Sonohysterogram. In this variation of ultrasound, saline is infused into the uterus to enhance visualization of the uterine cavity.

Treatment Options

When abnormal uterine bleeding is caused by internal changes in levels of estrogen and progesterone, it can often be regulated with prescription hormones, such as low-dose oral contraceptives. Other prescription hormonal drugs, such as progestogens, are also sometimes used for short-term treatment.

If nonsurgical treatments fail, several surgical procedures are available, depending on the cause of the abnormal bleeding (see box on page 12). If fibroids have been diagnosed, the decision to surgically remove them depends on their size, number, and location, as well as the severity of symptoms and a woman's desire for more children. Many of these procedures are used to remove fibroids, but they can also be used to evaluate and treat other kinds of abnormal uterine bleeding.

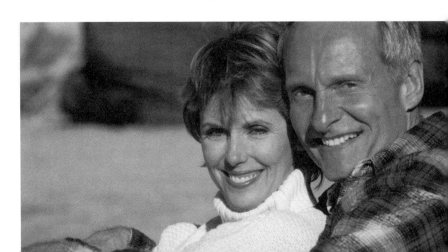

Surgical Procedures Often Used for Abnormal Uterine Bleeding

Laparoscopy. A tiny telescope (laparoscope) is inserted through a small incision in the abdomen. Pelvic organs can be viewed through the laparoscope and, sometimes, fibroids or cysts can be removed.

Operative hysteroscopy. A laser or electrical loop is inserted into the uterus through the cervix. Growths or polyps that bulge into the uterine cavity can be removed.

Endometrial ablation. The uterine lining is destroyed by freezing, heating, or cauterization, which ends fertility. Cannot be used when fibroids are the problem, unless the fibroids are also removed.

Dilation and curettage (D&C). Valuable in the past for determining the cause of abnormal uterine bleeding, but as a treatment, it seldom cures the condition of severe, consistent abnormal bleeding. Today, other surgical treatments are generally considered better options.

Abdominal myomectomy. Uses an abdominal incision to remove uterine fibroids (typically performed under general anesthesia).

Uterine artery embolization. Uses small plastic beads inserted into the uterine artery to block the blood flow to the fibroids, causing them to shrink. Indicated for women with fibroids who can't undergo surgery. Usually performed on an outpatient basis.

Hysterectomy. About 30% of all hysterectomies in the United States are performed for fibroids, and others are done for abnormal uterine bleeding. The uterus (and sometimes the cervix) is removed along with any fibroids that may be present. Afterward, pregnancy is no longer possible. The ovaries may or may not be removed (oophorectomy). If both ovaries are removed (bilateral oophorectomy), immediate surgical menopause occurs.

Bleeding After Menopause

Periods stop when a woman is past menopause, but taking some hormone treatments can cause bleeding to resume (see Progestogen & HRT). Unless the bleeding is the typical pattern caused by taking hormones, women who have uterine bleeding after menopause should see a clinician immediately to rule out serious causes, such as cancer.

HOT FLASHES

The most common perimenopausal discomfort is the hot flash (sometimes called hot flush). Hot flashes are the result of sudden changes in the body's "thermostat," the center of the brain that controls temperature regulation. If the brain's hypothalamus mistakenly senses that the woman is too warm,

it starts a chain of events to cool her down. Blood vessels near the surface of the skin begin to dilate so that blood rushes to the surface in an attempt to cool the body. This produces the red, flushed look to the face and neck. A woman may also begin to perspire so that the evaporating sweat can also cool the body. An increased pulse rate and a sensation of rapid heart beating may also occur. A cold chill often follows. A few women have only the chill.

Hot flashes that occur with drenching perspiration while sleeping are called night sweats. Night sweats and hot flashes may interfere with sleep, even if they are not strong enough to cause awakening. Also, falling estrogen levels alone can disrupt patterns of healthy deep sleep. While it is a myth that menopause itself makes a woman irritable, inadequate sleep causes fatigue, which may lead to irritability.

More than two-thirds of North American women have hot flashes during perimenopause. With induced menopause, almost all women have severe hot flashes that begin immediately following surgery or ovarian damage.

Hot flashes usually have a consistent pattern, but each woman's pattern is different. Some hot flashes are easily tolerated, others are annoying or embarrassing, and still others can be debilitating. Most women experience hot flashes for three to five years before they taper off. Although some women never have a hot flash or have them only for a few months, others may have them for many years. There is no way of knowing when they will stop.

Most women are able to identify particular triggers that seem to bring on their hot flashes, such as external heat (eg, a warm room or use of a hair dryer), strong emotions, hot drinks, hot or spicy foods, alcohol, and caffeine. A few drug therapies sometimes prescribed for women, such as tamoxifen (Nolvadex) for cancer chemotherapy and raloxifene (Evista) for prevention or treatment of osteoporosis, can cause hot flashes.

Treatment

Good news! There are many effective ways to relieve hot flashes, sometimes eliminating them entirely. They include the following:

- Avoid hot flash triggers;

- Keep cool by dressing in layers, using a fan, and sleeping in a cool room;

- Reduce stress by using meditation, yoga, biofeedback, visualization, massage, or a leisurely bath;

- Try paced respiration (deep, slow abdominal breathing) when a hot flash is starting;

- Exercise regularly to reduce stress and promote better, more restorative sleep.

Talk to a clinician about therapies available with or without a prescription.

Prescription estrogen replacement therapy is the standard medical treatment (see ERT). Considerable research has proven estrogen to be effective, and it is the only therapy approved by the FDA for treating hot flashes (see box below). Women should be reminded that having no treatment is an option, and hot flashes will typically stop on their own.

Other prescription drugs provide possible alternatives, but they are not well-proven or FDA-approved for this use. These include birth control pills, antihypertensives such as methyldopa (Aldomet) and clonidine (marketed as Catapres in the United States and Dixarit in Canada), antidepressants such as sertraline (Zoloft) and venlafaxine hydrochloride (Effexor), and

More than two-thirds of North American women have hot flashes during perimenopause.

What Does FDA Approval Mean?

In the prescription drug approval process, a manufacturer sends study information on a particular product to the US Food and Drug Administration (FDA). The FDA then considers the product's effectiveness, dosage, side effects, and possible risks. If FDA approval is given, the product may then be offered on the US market for the approved indication(s). All advertising and education from the manufacturer must comply with the FDA-approved prescribing information (package insert). Once a drug is on the market, clinicians can legally prescribe it for "off-label" (nonapproved) indications. An example would be using Catapres, a blood pressure medicine, to treat hot flashes.

a number of progestogens such as medroxyprogesterone acetate (Provera) and megestrol acetate (Megace).

Some women find relief from hot flashes by using remedies available over-the-counter (purchased without a prescription) at drugstores and health food stores. Black cohosh and isoflavones, such as those in soy and red clover, may help some women. Some of these remedies are often referred to as complementary and alternative medicine (CAM). Over-the-counter and CAM therapies may take two to six weeks before effects, if any, are felt (see Nonprescription Remedies; Complementary & Alternative Medicines). It is difficult to study how well these therapies work because placebo (dummy) medications relieve hot flashes in up to 40% of the women who take them.

> *There are many ways to relieve hot flashes.*

INSOMNIA

Some women experience menopause-related insomnia, especially if hormone changes provoke hot flashes. Sleep is adequate when one can function in an alert state during waking hours. Treatment of insomnia should first focus on improving sleep routine, such as avoiding heavy meals in the evening and adjusting levels of light, noise, and temperature. Avoiding alcohol, caffeine, and nicotine throughout the entire day (not just during the evening) can help increase sleep efficiency and total sleep time. Daily exercise can also help ease insomnia in many women, but exercising close to bedtime may have the opposite effect.

When lifestyle changes fail to alleviate sleep disturbances, a clinician should be consulted to discuss other options and to rule out disorders such as thyroid abnormalities, allergies, apnea (breathing problems), and anemia, which could be the culprit. Although estrogen is not FDA-approved for treatment of insomnia, ERT has been shown to improve sleep in some women (see ERT).

UROGENITAL CHANGES

During perimenopause, some women may begin to notice changes that occur in the urogenital area, which includes the vagina, genitals, and urinary tract. These urogenital changes can include the following:

- Dryness and/or irritation of the vagina;

- Itching and/or irritation of the vulva (outer genital area);

- Discomfort during sexual activity;

- Urgency or a more pressing need to urinate frequently;

- Urine leakage when coughing or sneezing.

These changes can range from mildly annoying to downright debilitating. There are many possible causes and effective treatments (see Menopause Treatment Options).

Vulvovaginal Problems

At some point in life, at least one-third of all women will experience some vulvovaginal problems, not all due to menopause. For example, an unusual vaginal discharge with an unpleasant odor or with itching and irritation of the vulva could be vaginitis, an inflammation of the vagina. While typically not a serious condition, vaginitis can be bothersome and sometimes recurrent. It sometimes resolves on its own. A clinician's diagnosis is essential to receiving proper treatment.

Other conditions that may cause vulvovaginal problems include:

- Vaginal infection, candidiasis (yeast fungus), and trichomoniasis;

- Bacterial vaginosis, an overgrowth of certain vaginal bacteria that causes a fishy odor and discharge;

- Sexually transmitted infections, including gonorrhea, chlamydia, or herpes, which may cause vaginal inflammation, discharge, pain, or itching;

- Skin diseases, such as eczema and Lichen sclerosus;

- Other diseases, such as Crohn's disease, an inflammatory bowel disorder;

- Pelvic radiation therapy, which can cause severe vaginal dryness and irritation;

- Medications, such as antibiotics, which can lead to a yeast infection; tamoxifen taken for breast cancer can cause an increase in vaginal discharge;

- Injury to pelvic nerve fibers, leading to persistent vulvar pain;

- Vulvodynia (pain in the vulva);

- Allergic reactions to chemicals in soaps, bubble baths, spermicides, condoms, feminine hygiene sprays, or deodorant tampons and pads;

- Irritation from tampons or birth control devices, such as a diaphragm or cervical cap, left inside the vagina too long;

- Douching (a practice that's not recommended).

In perimenopause and the years after menopause, many vulvovaginal changes can occur as a result of natural decreases in internal estrogen levels. This estrogen decline can cause tissues of the vulva and the lining of the vagina to become thin, dry, and less elastic – a condition known as atrophy. Over time, pubic hair becomes less abundant and vaginal walls become shorter and more narrow. Sometimes the vaginal lining becomes easily inflamed or broken, and may bleed. These vaginal tissues are also prone to injury during sexual relations or even a pelvic examination. Some factors that can place women at greater risk for vaginal atrophy include lack of regular sexual stimulation of the vagina, premature menopause, and history of temporary amenorrhea (missed periods). This lack of periods may be caused by extreme emotional distress, over-exercising, or over-dieting during the reproductive years, resulting in an underlying problem of low estrogen.

If the thin, alkaline vagina becomes inflamed, it is called atrophic vaginitis. This type of vaginitis is not an infection. However, without treatment, the vaginal lining may deteriorate to a thickness of only a few cell layers, and small vaginal ulcers can occur. In fact, vaginal pain and bleeding during sexual intercourse can intensify to the point where intercourse is no longer pleasurable or possible.

Women near or beyond menopause should not assume that vulvovaginal problems are due to reduced estrogen levels. All vulvovaginal changes should be investigated by a clinician to determine the true cause.

Treatment. Vaginal lubricants and moisturizers available without a prescription may help in milder cases of vaginal atrophy (see Nonprescription Remedies). Regular sexual activity has also been shown to maintain vaginal health. If these measures are ineffective, then the best treatment is to use supplemental estrogen.

Prescription estrogen therapy quickly restores the thickness and elasticity of these tissues and also relieves vaginal dryness. All dosage forms are effective and FDA-approved for this use, but vaginal atrophy symptoms may respond more quickly to the vaginal forms of estrogen (vaginal creams, vaginal tablet, and vaginal ring). In cases of severe vaginal atrophy, several weeks of treatment may be required to restore the vagina to a healthy condition.

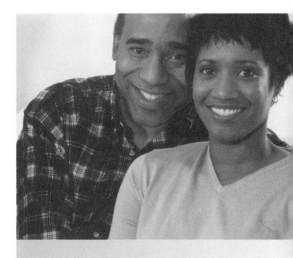

Regular sexual activity can help maintain vaginal health.

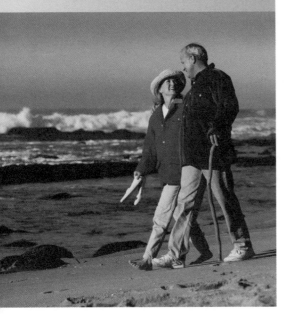

Incontinence is not an inevitable result of aging.

A diet enriched with soy foods (which contain plant estrogens) may help reduce vaginal discomfort for some women, although an improvement may not be observed for weeks (see Complementary & Alternative Medicines).

Urinary Conditions

As menopause approaches and during the years that follow, lack of estrogen can cause the lining of the urethra, the outlet for the bladder, to become thin. With aging, the surrounding pelvic muscles may weaken. As a result, a woman may have one or more of the following urinary conditions:

- Frequency – the need to urinate more often;

- Urgency – a sudden need to urinate even though the bladder may not be full;

- Nocturia – a need to get out of bed to urinate several times during the night;

- Stress incontinence – urine leakage upon coughing, laughing, sneezing, or lifting;

- Painful urination.

When urine leakage and lack of bladder control become so problematic they have an impact on hygiene and/or overall well-being, the condition is called urinary incontinence. While incontinence can occur at any time, the likelihood of becoming incontinent increases with age because of a variety of factors, including decreasing estrogen. Other possible contributing factors to urinary incontinence are the following:

- Cystitis or infections of the bladder;

- Urethritis or infections of the urethra;

- Weakening of the pelvic muscles and ligaments due to natural aging or previous damage from childbirth injury;

- Certain prescription drugs, such as diuretics and some tranquilizers;

- Irritated bladder caused by smoking cigarettes, drinking alcohol and/or caffeine;

- Other medical conditions, such as the nerve disorder multiple sclerosis.

Although up to 40% of women aged 45 to 64 have urinary incontinence, less than half seek help. This is often because of embarrassment or the misconception that the condition is a normal part of aging and cannot be treated. In reality, diagnosis and treatment can often completely cure the problem. If a cure is not possible, comfort can usually be improved. Incontinence should never be viewed as an inevitable result of aging.

To diagnose the exact cause(s) of incontinence, a clinician obtains a medical and sexual history, and performs a physical examination, including a pelvic exam and analysis of a urine sample. Keeping a voiding diary can be helpful (see box on page 17). Additional specialized studies of the bladder are often needed.

Treatment. Today, there are many options to treat urinary incontinence, and more are in development. The best option, however, depends on the cause of incontinence. Treatment options include the following:

Kegel exercises consist of repeated contraction and relaxation of the urogenital muscles, toning the muscles that control urine flow. When done correctly, Kegels are highly effective but must be continued indefinitely. Another potential benefit is improvement of vaginal sexual function.

Prescription medications, such as certain anticholinergic drugs (Detrol, Ditropan) that control abnormal bladder contractions, are FDA-approved for the treatment of incontinence. Estrogen therapy, although not FDA-approved for this use, has been reported to produce improvement in some women with certain types of incontinence, but the evidence is weak. Estrogen may also help reduce the risk of urinary tract infection. Urinary tract infections or infections of the vaginal area brought on by urine leakage are treated with antibiotics.

Devices, such as a pessary (inserted into the vagina to support the uterus or bladder) or those used to block the urethra, can relieve incontinence for some women.

Biofeedback with electrical stimulation of muscles is used to help retrain the bladder.

Surgery is used to correct anatomical defects.

When urinary incontinence does not improve with initial treatment, a physician with expertise in female urology or urogynecology should be consulted. A specialist is also recommended when there is a complex condition, such as a neurologic disease or when surgery is being considered.

CHANGES IN SEXUAL FUNCTION

Sexuality is a natural part of living, and sexual feelings, desires, and activities are healthy throughout life.

In fact, many women remain sexually active well into older age.

Sexual concerns are common in midlife women. As mentioned earlier, changes in the vagina brought on by falling estrogen levels at menopause can make intercourse painful. In addition, it is not unusual for male partners to experience sexual problems, including impotence, as they age.

Sexual desire (libido) is also an important component of sexual function, and it decreases with age for both sexes. Many women during their 40s and 50s notice they have less sexual desire, but exactly how menopause and hormones may contribute to this change is unknown.

No correlation has been found between falling estrogen levels and declining libido. Androgen, however, does appear to play a role in women's sex drive, and aging ovaries also produce less androgen, although the decline is not so steep as with estrogen.

The conditions that further decrease internal androgen levels include surgical removal of one or both ovaries prior to menopause, pituitary and adrenal insufficiency, corticosteroid therapy, and chronic illness. Treatments are available for some of these sexual function problems.

Advice For Women With Urinary Conditions

Keeping a voiding (urination) diary for one week will help establish voiding patterns, the first step in determining the cause of the problem. Each day, record the following:

- Type and amount of fluid intake and time of day

- Amount of urine voided and time of day

- Any urge that was sensed before voiding

- Amount of urine leaked, whether it was just a few drops or wet underwear or soaked clothing

- Time of day and type of activity when the leakage occurred

Numerous factors influence a woman's sexual activity and interest during midlife and later, including the following:

Previous attitudes often dictate a woman's view of her sexuality as she ages. In general, women who enjoyed sex in their younger years continue to do so during and beyond midlife. Those who did not enjoy sex previously may view any midlife reduction in sexual activity as relief rather than loss. Partners may also lose interest in sex or have decreased capacity for sexual activity. Some women, however, have an increased interest in sex.

Many women remain sexually active well into older age.

Age-related changes can affect sexual functioning. Although sexual desire generally decreases in both men and women over time, a decline does not mean an abrupt halt, and the rate and extent of any decline is individual.

A woman's perception of her body is an important component of her sexual health. Menopause usually occurs at a time when women are experiencing changes in physical appearance. A woman who accepts her changing body and maintains a positive outlook about it is more comfortable with herself and tends to experience greater sexual enjoyment. Partners, too, are typically changing in their appearance, and this can also affect sexual encounters.

Health concerns of both women and men, such as the pain and fear associated with serious illnesses, can significantly interfere with mutual enjoyment of sexual relations. A woman may feel unattractive and may avoid initiating sexual encounters after a surgical procedure, such as removal of a breast or the uterus. Likewise, her partner may avoid intercourse, fearing that vaginal penetration will cause her pain.

Incontinence can lead to sexual avoidance.

Sleep disturbances from hot flashes at night can make a woman tired and irritable, thereby affecting sexual desire.

Depression, stress and anxiety may have an impact on a woman's primary erogenous zone – her brain – undermining sexual desire.

Many medications, such as those for high blood pressure and depression, can create problems with sexual desire and orgasmic capacity.

Induced menopause can lessen sexual desire.

Sexual Function Issues

The following are issues that may be important when discussing sexual function with a clinician:

Types of sexual relations

Types of sexual activities

Status of relationship

Number of sexual partners past and present

Sexual orientation

Habits related to self-stimulation

Ability to achieve orgasm

Changes in sexual interest

Changes in arousal

Adherence to safer sex practices

History of STIs and testing for STIs

Birth control method(s) used

Satisfaction level with current sex life

Medications and remedies used, both prescription and nonprescription

Hysterectomy can affect sexual function, and women and their partners need reassurance that losing the uterus does not mean losing sexual desire and femininity. During intercourse and orgasm, some women may notice a change in sensation after hysterectomy, but in general, these changes do not interfere with sexual functioning or achieving orgasm. In fact, many women have improved sex lives after hysterectomy due to relief from pain and bleeding, and the lack of need for birth control.

Treatment

The hectic pace of life can interfere with emotional and physical intimacy, and couples can take their sex lives for granted. Good communication is the key for understanding sexual changes. Some couples find that intercourse takes more time or they fail to make time for quality sexual encounters.

Men may experience a lack of sexual interest or difficulty achieving erection or ejaculation, and may need more manual or oral stimulation of the penis. Women, too, may need more stimulation to achieve adequate lubrication or orgasm.

Intercourse does not have to be the primary sexual activity. More attention can be devoted to other sexual behaviors that may be as satisfying, such as oral sex, massage, sensual baths, manual stimulation, and caressing. Women without partners can explore masturbation, a normal and healthy expression of sexual interest. Using a vibrator or dildo may enhance sexual pleasure.

Understanding these factors, making adjustments, and getting any necessary medical treatments can alleviate anxiety and improve sexual activity. It is a myth that sex education is only for the young. An individual's sexual function changes with age, and a need for information accompanies these changes.

While many women find it difficult to discuss the intimate aspects of their sexual relations, healthcare providers are better able to help them achieve optimal sexual health after an open discussion on sexual history and lifestyle. If needed, a referral to a specialist in sexual counseling can be provided.

Drug therapy to improve sexual function is a field still in its infancy, and many studies are being conducted. A small number of studies have produced conflicting results on estrogen's ability to improve sexual drive or arousal. Estrogen probably does not improve sex drive independent of making intercourse less painful by treating atrophy of the vagina. However, adding androgen to estrogen therapy may be helpful in boosting libido (see Prescription Therapies). Other prescription therapies and over-the-counter products advertised to improve female or male sexual function

> *The risk of sexually transmitted infections, including AIDS, is a lifelong concern.*

Safer Sex Guidelines

Discuss sexual history with a potential sex partner; don't let embarrassment compromise health.

Always insist that male partners use a latex condom for genital, oral, and anal sex unless in a long-standing, mutually monogamous relationship; never use petroleum-based oils such as Vaseline or baby oil for lubrication because they can damage condoms.

Choose sex partners selectively.

Keep medically fit by having an annual physical exam, a Pap test when indicated, and tests to identify STIs.

Urge any partner exposed to an STI or with a confirmed diagnosis to be examined and treated.

are not recommended for women due to lack of data on safety and effectiveness.

Protection Is Essential

The risk of pregnancy is eliminated only after menopause has been reached (see Birth Control As Menopause Approaches). But protection from pregnancy is not necessarily protection against sexually transmitted infections (STIs). The risk of STIs, including syphilis, chlamydia, gonorrhea, genital herpes, genital warts, hepatitis B, and HIV (the AIDS virus), is a lifelong concern for sexually active women. In fact, postmenopausal women without adequate estrogen levels may be at increased risk for STIs. Delicate vaginal tissue, prone to small tears and cuts, can act as pathways for infection.

Safer sex guidelines (see box on page 19) are important even if a woman has had a hysterectomy or her ovaries removed. Most STIs are more easily transmitted to women than to men. STIs are also less likely to produce symptoms in women, making them more difficult to diagnose until serious problems develop.

PSYCHOLOGICAL CHANGES

There are many myths associated with menopause. One is the myth that mental health problems, such as depression and anxiety, are inevitable as hormone production decreases. In reality, there are no scientific studies to support the belief that natural menopause contributes to true clinical depression, anxiety, severe memory lapses, or erratic behavior.

However, many midlife women do suffer from feeling blue or discouraged. Others suffer from sleep deprivation and overwork, leading to fatigue and sometimes irritability. Support and encouragement can help women find their way through any difficult time to thrive once again during what can be the best years of their lives.

During reproductive years, most women become accustomed to their own hormonal rhythm, but during perimenopause, this rhythm changes.

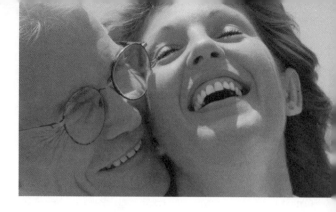

These hormonal fluctuations, although normal, can contribute to mood swings. The unexpected timing of menopause can also be upsetting. For some, the hormone-related changes coincide with other stressors and losses in life. Women in midlife are not unaccustomed to stress, but some women can be especially vulnerable to stressors that may arise. Potential sources of midlife stress include:

- Floundering relationships;

- Divorce or widowhood;

- Care of young children, struggles with adolescents, or return of grown children to the home;

- Being childless, sometimes not by choice;

- Concerns about aging parents, caregiving responsibilities;

- Career and education issues;

- Body changes with aging.

In addition, in today's youth-valued society, getting older can be difficult. Midlife women often experience changes in self-concept, self-esteem, and body image. They may start to think about their own mortality and become introspective about the meaning or purpose of their lives.

Although these changes can be opportunities for positive transformation and growth, some women react by feeling overwhelmed, out of control, angry, and/or numb. They may look for refuge in alcohol or drugs and, thus, compound their problems.

In fact, women are more likely than men to drink more in response to feeling blue, experiencing loss or divorce, or children leaving home. Thus, although not caused by menopause, psychological problems can arise during midlife.

Creating Balance

Emotional health during perimenopause requires a balance between self-nurturing and the obligations of work and caring for others. Many women are able to identify and describe sources of tension and symptoms of stress, but they often find it difficult to take care of themselves during these times.

Recognizing a problem can lead to understanding its causes and developing new coping mechanisms. Although many stressors cannot be altered, coping skills can be learned to make a woman feel empowered to meet life's challenges. A renewed sense of self-confidence can restore balance and harmony (see box below).

Ruling Out Disease

Sometimes, coping skills are not sufficient to relieve the symptoms of stress. These feelings may be a side effect of medication, a symptom of a medical condition, or the result of depression. A healthcare provider can help determine the cause of mental health stressors, assess options, and prescribe appropriate treatment.

Treatment

The psychological disturbances reported most often by perimenopausal women are irritability and blue moods. These can often be relieved through lifestyle changes. Relaxation and stress-reduction techniques help many women cope with life stress factors during this time of hormonal fluctuation. Mood disturbances brought on by sleep deprivation resulting from hot flashes usually improve when hot flashes are treated.

Clinical depression is not related to menopause, but it is associated with a chemical imbalance in the brain. If medication is needed for mild to moderate depression, herbal remedies such as St. John's wort may help (see Complementary & Alternative Medicines). If the depression is more severe, one of a variety of effective prescription antidepressant medications can be prescribed to correct the chemical imbalance. Although several weeks are usually needed for the drug's full effect, most women show a marked improvement with these medications with relatively few side effects. Antidepressant medication is best used in combination with counseling or psychotherapy.

> *Balance and harmony can be achieved along with an all-important sense of self-confidence.*

Beating Stress

Participate in pleasurable activities

Talk with friends

Make time for regular, daily exercise

Find or renew a creative outlet or activity that fulfills mental and spiritual needs

Enjoy activities such as a massage or manicure

Eat three nutritious meals a day, don't skip meals

Snack on healthful, crunchy foods, such as apples and raw carrots

Try stress reduction and relaxation techniques, such as deep breathing and meditation

Get adequate sleep each night

Laugh as much as possible

Hormone therapy, as part of a comprehensive treatment plan, is reported to help some women with depression. Many women respond well to estrogen therapy, but it may actually worsen mood in some women who are clinically depressed. The prescription hormone progestin, a synthetic progestogen, may also worsen mood, particularly in a woman with a history of mood changes prior to each menstrual period during younger years. Women who must take progestin to protect the uterus from cancer and who have mood problems while taking one drug regimen may find relief by trying different forms, doses, or regimens of progestogens. No hormone is FDA-approved for relief of psychological symptoms.

Anxiety

Anxiety – an agitated sense of anticipation, dread, or fear – is experienced by everyone at one time or another. Perimenopausal women may have more anxiety due to physical and psychological changes as well as a variety of stressors. Although this anxiety usually resolves on its own without treatment, it may accompany or be a warning sign of another medical illness, such as panic disorder.

Panic disorder can result in shortness of breath, chest pain, dizziness, heart palpitations, and/or feelings of "going crazy" or being out of control. Sometimes the unsettling feelings that precede a hot flash can trigger feelings of panic or an attack of anxiety. Sometimes anxiety symptoms can be related to depression.

Women with severe symptoms of anxiety can usually find relief through therapeutic approaches, including prescription drug treatment, relaxation techniques, stress reduction techniques, counseling, and psychotherapy.

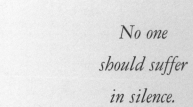

No one should suffer in silence.

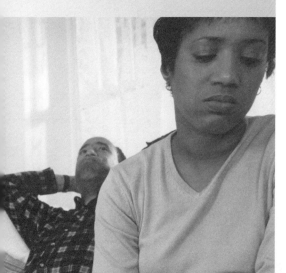

Concentration & Memory

Perimenopausal women frequently report difficulty concentrating and minor memory problems (especially remembering something that was very recent). These difficulties often frighten women, who may think they are beginning to have early symptoms of Alzheimer's disease. This is rarely the case. More research is needed to determine the cause of these complaints. They may be more related to stress and aging than to the menopause transition. Some women report that estrogen therapy provides relief, but estrogen is not FDA-approved for this use. Also, lowered estrogen levels may be associated with memory problems and Alzheimer's disease later in life, although research in this area is contradictory.

Seeking Help

Although some individuals may feel embarrassed or even ashamed about revealing their mental health problems, no one should suffer in silence. Women should seek help from their healthcare provider, who will be better able to help when given as many facts as possible about family and personal history.

Most healthcare providers are not specifically trained in the management of mental health disorders. A consultation with a mental health professional is sometimes appropriate. For a specific problem, such as marital trouble or an eating disorder, a counselor with expertise in that area is best. Consultation with a mental health professional is not a commitment to long-term treatment, and getting an expert opinion can be reassuring.

OTHER HEALTH CHANGES

Perimenopausal women often report other health changes that may or may not be attributed to approaching menopause. Among these changes are weight gain, heart palpitations, joint pain, headache, and changes in the skin, eyes, hair, and teeth.

Weight Gain

In their 40s and 50s, women often gain weight and sometimes attribute this gain to menopause or hormone therapy for menopause-related conditions. However, the notion that menopause or hormone therapy is responsible for weight gain is not supported by scientific evidence. Midlife weight gain appears to be mostly related to aging and lifestyle. Studies reveal the following:

- Behavioral factors, particularly decreased exercise and increased alcohol consumption, are more closely linked to weight gain than either menopause or hormone therapy.

- Body shape typically changes with aging – from a "pear" (wide hips and thighs) to an "apple" (wide waist).

- Muscle mass often decreases, while fat often increases. Although this shift may not increase weight (muscle weighs more than fat), body size will go up. The loss of muscle mass also decreases metabolic rate and lowers a woman's caloric need, which can lead to weight gain.

Exercise seems to have the most beneficial effect on minimizing fat increases and maintaining muscle (thereby minimizing body size and increasing caloric need). Women, both perimenopausal and postmenopausal, who are looking for a lower fat-to-muscle ratio will find more reward in resistance-type exercises, such as weight lifting.

In general, fewer calories are needed after menopause, when less energy is expended. Thus, a woman can eat the same amount and gain weight.

Heart Palpitations

There is no scientific evidence linking heart rhythm abnormalities (palpitations) with the diminished hormone levels of menopause. However, an increase of 8 to 16 beats in heart rate can occur during a hot flash, which some women may interpret as a heart problem. Palpitations may also be the result of thyroid disease or anxiety experienced with mood changes or from more serious psychological upset. It is unlikely that palpitations experienced at this time are related to heart disease. Nevertheless, women experiencing heart palpitations should report these feelings to their healthcare provider to rule out serious illness.

Joint Pain

There are no studies linking menopause and joint pain. However, the risk of osteoarthritis – the most common form of joint disease – increases with aging. Suffering from joint pain is not inevitable. A woman's healthcare provider can recommend the best type of exercises to help alleviate pain and, if needed, over-the-counter and prescription therapies.

Headache

Studies suggest that perimenopausal hormonal fluctuations may play a role in headaches. Women at special risk for hormonal headaches during perimenopause are those sensitive to hormone fluctuations, which is usually indicated by a history of headaches at the same time each month during their menstruating years. Some non-hormonal causes of headaches are infection, dental

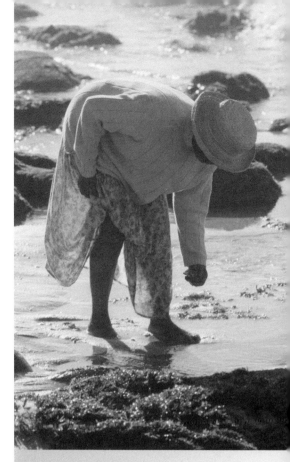

There are no scientific studies to support the belief that natural menopause is responsible for clinical depression, anxiety, severe memory lapses, or erratic behavior.

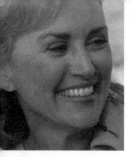

problems, or sinus problems, and some can be a sign of more serious conditions, such as hypertension.

Most headaches are minor, but some can be more severe and interfere with daily life. These include the following:

- Tension headaches – Squeezing or pressing pain across the forehead or around the head that often occurs upon waking; the headache can last from 30 minutes to several days.

- Migraine headaches – Severe, throbbing pain, typically located one-sided at the temple, that occurs periodically; the headache may be accompanied by nausea, vomiting, and sensitivity to light and noise.

- Cluster headaches – Multiple episodes of short-lived but severe one-sided pain.

Most headaches either do not require treatment or can be treated with nonprescription pain medications. Hormonal headaches that are related to hormone fluctuations of perimenopause can sometimes be relieved through hormone therapy that attempts to level the fluctuations. With migraine headaches, estrogen may either make them better or worse. Estrogen is not FDA-approved for treatment of headaches, but there are several other prescription drugs approved for this use.

Skin Changes

The skin undergoes normal changes with aging, including loss of collagen and elasticity, creating slight sags and wrinkles. Skin becomes more dry and flaky. Drinking plenty of water and using skin creams will help keep skin moisturized. Long-time smokers have even greater skin damage, particularly wrinkles around the lips and dark circles under the eyes. Maintaining skin health is yet another reason not to smoke.

Aging skin becomes more prone to sun damage, so protecting the skin from harmful UV rays

through use of a good sunscreen is more important than ever. Any dark or changing moles should be evaluated by a clinician.

A small percentage of perimenopausal women report irritating sensations to the skin, ranging from severe itching to phantom symptoms of "ants crawling under their skin." This condition, called formication (from the Greek word for ant), is difficult to diagnose and even more difficult to treat. There are no scientific studies to guide clinicians. Sometimes hormone therapy or antihistamines will help.

Hair Changes

Getting older increases the likelihood for hair to become gray and more brittle. In addition, excessive hair growth can occur in areas of the body where hair follicles are most androgen-sensitive, such as the chin, upper lip, and cheeks. Women often report a large "rogue hair" on their chin that seems to grow to a great length almost overnight. Hair thinning may also occur, a condition that is typically genetic and in response to a shift in the internal balance between estrogen and androgen. After menopause, the increase in the androgen-to-estrogen ratio may cause hair thinning to worsen.

However, the tendency for hair thinning may decrease for women experiencing surgical menopause because the internal androgen levels plummet after the ovaries are removed. Androgen therapy may result in hair loss; some women also have hair loss with estrogen therapy.

Eating a healthy diet, adding a daily multivitamin, and avoiding harsh chemicals and sunlight that dry the hair will help keep hair healthy. Treating severe hair loss is more of a challenge because finding the cause is often difficult. Women suffering from this condition should consult a dermatologist.

Eye Changes

Aging often results in the need to wear corrective lenses. There is also an increased risk of eye diseases such as cataracts and macular degeneration. Some women report dryness, scratchiness, and burning of the eyes, as well as light and cold intolerance. Use of eye moisturizers can help for this dry eye syndrome. If symptoms persist, an ophthalmologist should be consulted.

Dental Changes

After menopause, there is an increase in tooth loss, the need for dentures, and gingival bleeding and inflammation. Thus, good dental hygiene and regular checkups are as important as ever. Some dental changes may be related to diminished levels of internal estrogen. Often, tooth loss is a sign of underlying bone disease, such as osteoporosis. A woman's primary healthcare provider needs to be kept current on any changes observed by her dentist.

When midlife women move beyond menopause into postmenopause, they may experience changes due to aging that may or may not be related to declining hormone levels. These changes include serious health conditions such as heart disease, osteoporosis, and cancer. Risks for developing these are best determined as early as possible, so that preventive strategies can be employed.

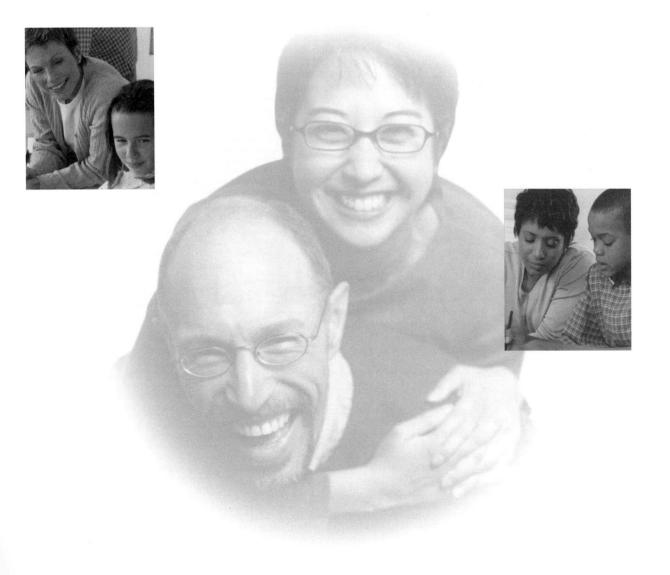

POSTMENOPAUSAL
HEALTH

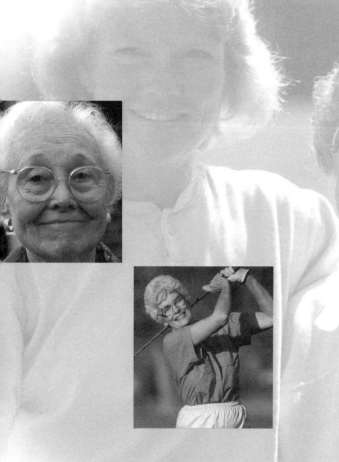

MOST WOMEN WHO READ THIS

BOOKLET ARE INTERESTED IN THE ISSUES

SURROUNDING PERIMENOPAUSE.

HOWEVER, POSTMENOPAUSE MUST BE

UNDERSTOOD AS WELL. DECISIONS MADE

AT PERIMENOPAUSE OR WHEN INDUCED

MENOPAUSE OCCURS AFFECT A WOMAN'S

HEALTH FOR THE REST OF HER LIFE.

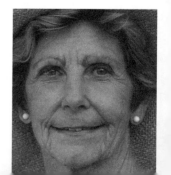

When midlife women move beyond menopause into postmenopause, they may experience changes due to aging that may or may not be related to declining hormone levels. These changes include serious health conditions such as heart disease, osteoporosis, and cancer. Risks for developing these are best determined as early as possible, so that preventive strategies can be employed.

HEART DISEASE

Many women think of heart disease as a man's disease. In reality, heart disease is the number-one killer of women in North America. After age 50, nearly half of all deaths in women are caused by some form of cardiovascular disease. Nearly twice as many women die from heart disease as die from breast cancer. It is speculated that estrogen protects women from heart disease. While a man's risk of heart disease starts to increase significantly after age 45, women begin to be more at risk after menopause, when estrogen levels fall.

Studies have identified several factors that increase a woman's risk of heart disease (see box). The higher the risk of heart disease, the more aggressive the prevention strategy should be.

Heart disease and cardiovascular disease are umbrella terms used to describe many conditions related to the circulatory system, inside and outside the heart. Heart health refers to health of the entire cardiovascular system, not just the heart itself.

Coronary arteries supply the heart muscle with nutrients and oxygen. Coronary heart disease (sometimes called coronary artery disease) refers to damaged or diseased blood vessels inside the heart. The most common form of heart disease, it is caused by the build-up of substances called plaque in the lining of coronary blood vessels, causing reduced blood flow. When one of these arteries is completely blocked, a heart attack occurs. Heart disease is often detected later in women than in men because women's symptoms can be different. Confusion also exists because chest pain without heart disease is very common in younger women. However, as women age, chest pain is more likely to be related to heart disease.

Outside the heart, diseased blood vessels can cause adverse conditions, such as stroke, high blood pressure, and poor circulation, which can lead to difficulty walking and even to loss of limbs.

Maintaining Heart Health

While some risk factors cannot be changed, others can be controlled or modified to create a more heart-healthy lifestyle, including the following:

Don't smoke. Of all the lifestyle factors that can be changed, smoking cessation has the

Heart Disease Risk Factors

Advancing age

Black race

Cigarette smoking

Physical inactivity

High blood pressure

Abnormal cholesterol levels

Stress

Diabetes

Drinking more than three alcoholic beverages daily

Family history: A close blood relative who had a stroke; a father or brother who had a heart attack before age 55; a mother or sister who had a heart attack before age 65

Weight more than 30% over ideal

Past menopause, especially if reached before 40

greatest impact on saving lives. Smokers are considerably more likely to have a heart attack than nonsmokers. But there's good news. When a woman stops smoking, no matter how long or how much she smoked, her risk of heart disease drops by 50% the first year. There are many other good reasons not to smoke, including increased vitality, improved appearance, and decreased risk of lung disease.

Get regular exercise. A sedentary lifestyle of physical inactivity is almost as great a risk factor for heart disease as smoking because of diminished circulation and weight gain.

Maintain healthy weight. Even with no other risk factors, being more than 30% overweight places a woman at risk for heart disease.

> *A sedentary lifestyle is almost as great a risk factor for heart disease as smoking.*

Reduce stress. A stressful lifestyle increases risk of heart disease and many other health problems. Exercise, meditation, and relaxation techniques can significantly reduce stress.

Control blood pressure. High blood pressure (hypertension) is defined as an arm cuff reading greater than 140/90 mm Hg, although it is preferable to keep blood pressure below that level. Even mild elevations can double the risk of stroke or heart attack. High blood pressure becomes more common with aging. In fact, more than half of all women over age 65 are affected. Black women are especially susceptible. Regular testing is important because high blood pressure rarely causes symptoms. Although it cannot be cured, high blood pressure can be controlled by eating a healthy diet, limiting the intake of salt and alcohol, exercising on a regular basis, and reducing stress. Controlling weight is also important; losing just 5 to 10 pounds often brings blood pressure down to normal. If these

measures fail to control blood pressure, several prescription medications are available to enhance the beneficial effects of these lifestyle modifications.

Control cholesterol. Abnormal blood levels of cholesterol can cause a build-up of fatty deposits on the inner walls of the arteries that supply blood to the heart and the rest of the body. This is called atherosclerosis or hardening of the arteries. The fatty deposits slow down blood flow and can block the vessel entirely. If this happens to a blood vessel in the brain, a stroke can occur. If it happens to a blood vessel in the heart, a heart attack can occur.

More than one-third of all women have cholesterol levels that put them at increased risk for heart disease. Bringing cholesterol levels to within normal limits has an enormous impact on heart disease risk. Total cholesterol should be less than 200 mg/dL (5.17 mmol/L). Other goals include maintaining high levels of high-density lipoprotein cholesterol (HDL-C, the "good cholesterol") and low levels of low-density lipoprotein cholesterol (LDL-C, the "bad cholesterol"). Target levels for HDL-C are at least 35 mg/dL (0.91 mmol/L); for LDL-C, they are less than 130 mg/day (3.36 mmol/L) or less than 100 mg/dL (2.59 mmol/L) for women with known heart disease or diabetes.

Cholesterol-healthy tips include eating food with little or no cholesterol and animal fat, choosing olive or canola oil for cooking, and avoiding hydrogenated oil and trans-fatty acids found in foods such as margarine and prepared foods with a long shelf-life. Exercising on a regular basis and controlling weight are also beneficial. When diet and exercise aren't enough, special cholesterol-lowering prescription medications are available. Estrogen therapy can also increase HDL and lower LDL, although the role of prescription estrogen in preventing heart disease has not been definitively determined.

Control triglycerides. Most fats in the blood exist as triglycerides. A healthy level of less than 200 mg/dL (5.17 mmol/L) can usually be maintained through not smoking, limiting alcohol intake, avoiding food with fat and sugar, exercising regularly, and keeping weight under control. Preventing diabetes (or keeping it under control) is also important.

Prevent diabetes. High levels of blood sugar (diabetes) increase the risk of cardiovascular disease. Women with diabetes have a two to three times higher risk of heart attack than women without diabetes and have twice the risk of a second heart attack. Midlife women should be screened for diabetes if they are at high risk (family history of diabetes, obesity, personal history of gestational diabetes, or member of a high-risk ethnic group).

Diet, exercise, and weight control are especially important for any woman with diabetes or at high risk for diabetes. Medication may also be needed to control blood sugar. If a woman with diabetes needs hormone therapy for menopause-related conditions, an estrogen skin patch may be a better choice than an estrogen pill. For uterine protection, a better choice may be using progesterone instead of synthetic progestin. Androgen therapy should be avoided (see Prescription Therapies).

The Effect of Menopause

When menopause is reached and estrogen levels drop, the risk for heart disease increases. The coronary heart disease rates in postmenopausal women are two to three times higher than those in premenopausal women the same age. Thus, a careful assessment of a woman's heart disease risk factors is very important at this time. Women who experience premature menopause, natural or induced, are probably at even greater risk for heart disease.

Treatment Options

In addition to altering lifestyle, there are many FDA-approved prescription medications to help control specific conditions, such as high blood pressure (eg, diuretics) and cholesterol (eg, statins).

Although not FDA-approved for this use, estrogen therapy has been shown in some studies to reduce the risk of heart disease, but its role in preventing heart disease remains to be clarified. Estrogen definitely raises HDL and lowers LDL, and it has other good effects, such as relaxing the smooth muscle in the blood vessels, helping to keep them open.

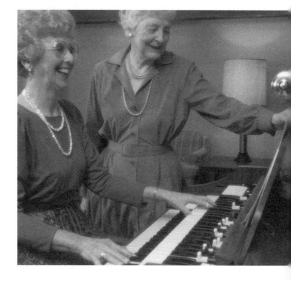

Some recent evidence suggests that estrogen therapy increases the risk for blood-clotting disorders, including blocking of the main blood vessels in the lung (pulmonary embolism). Raloxifene (Evista), used for osteoporosis, can also increase blood clot risks. Although these disorders are rare, women with a tendency toward forming blood clots may not be candidates for therapy with estrogen or raloxifene.

Nonprescription products are also used by many women to lower their risk of heart disease. Studies have found daily low-dose (baby) aspirin to be effective. Vitamin E, once thought to lower risk, has been proven ineffective. Folate as well as soy foods and supplements are still being studied.

OSTEOPOROSIS

Postmenopausal osteoporosis is a disease in which the bone mineral content of the skeleton gradually decreases with age until the bone has become fragile and susceptible to fractures. Tiny fractures of the spine are the most frequent type of osteoporotic fracture, and they may lead to chronic back pain, loss of height, and curvature of the upper back. Having had one spine fracture substantially increases the risk for subsequent fractures. Hip fractures, although not as frequent as spine fractures, are more serious. Between 10% and 15% of hip-fracture victims die within one year of their fracture (typically from pneumonia due to lack of mobility), with about one-third becoming permanent nursing home residents. Only about half of the survivors are able to return to fully independent living.

Bones grow during childhood and adolescence, reaching their strongest point (peak bone mass) between the ages of 20 and 30. From then on, bone loss occurs gradually for the remainder of life. In most women, bone loss accelerates during the first few years after menopause, which is related to the decline in estrogen levels that occurs at that time.

Osteoporosis can be caused by an inadequate amount of bone made during growth years or by an increased rate of bone loss in adulthood – or both. Major risk factors that increase vulnerability to osteoporosis are presented in the box below.

Detecting Osteoporosis

Early detection of bone loss can lead to treatment that may restore lost bone mass and help reduce the chance of fracture. Osteoporosis has no early warning signs, so it is not usually detected until it has become advanced. Prolonged and severe pain in the middle of the back and tooth loss are two possible indicators of underlying bone loss. Other signs are changes in the shape of the spine and loss of height. While it's normal to lose some height while aging, most experts agree that a loss of two inches or more is cause for concern. Standard x-rays are not sensitive enough to reveal osteoporosis until a considerable amount of bone has already been lost. Among the tests used to detect osteoporosis are the following:

Bone density testing. Measuring bone density is the best way to evaluate bone strength. Today, bone mineral density (BMD) is measured in ways that are not only more accurate than standard x-ray, but also safe and painless. Dual-energy x-ray absorptiometry (DEXA) is the preferred technology. It measures spine, hip, or total body BMD, providing reliability while using only 10% of the radiation in a chest x-ray. DEXA can be used to determine the presence and severity of osteoporosis, to predict the risk of developing osteoporosis, and to monitor the effects of treatments.

Ultrasound, which does not require radiation, is used to measure bone density in peripheral body sites, such as the wrist or heel. Ultrasound measurements can be used to predict fracture risk; however, they cannot be used to make the diagnosis of osteoporosis or to monitor the effects of therapy.

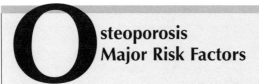

Osteoporosis Major Risk Factors

Advanced age

Caucasian or Asian race

Female gender

Family history of osteoporosis

Small boned and/or thin

Sedentary lifestyle

Lack of adequate calcium and vitamin D

Absence of menstrual periods during the reproductive years for longer than six months (excluding pregnancy)

Use of certain bone-robbing prescription medicines, such as steroids and antiseizure drugs

Thyroid disease, with excessive doses of thyroid medication

Past menopause, especially if premature

Blood and urine tests. Throughout life, bone is constantly renewed, with old bone being removed and new bone being formed – a process called bone remodeling. Lab tests can measure bone breakdown products in the blood and urine. Although these measurements are not used for diagnosis of osteoporosis, they may be useful in monitoring response to osteoporosis treatment.

Prevention & Treatment

The primary goal of osteoporosis therapy is to prevent fractures by stopping or slowing loss of bone mass, maintaining bone strength, and minimizing or eliminating factors that contribute to falls.

Maintaining a healthy lifestyle, including regular weight-bearing exercise and an adequate intake of calcium and vitamin D, is a preventive measure that is believed to help slow bone loss in the early postmenopausal years and reduce fracture risk in older women. Although lifestyle measures do not work as well as prescription therapies, they will enhance the positive effects of the drugs. The following are the primary prescription therapies available for osteoporosis management:

ERT/HRT. Estrogen (as estrogen replacement therapy or ERT) is a proven therapy for reducing the incidence of osteoporosis associated with menopause. Studies have shown that ERT prevents bone loss in women who begin therapy soon after menopause. Estrogen increases bone mass in women over the age of 60 and is thought to decrease the frequency of fractures, primarily spine fractures. Formal studies documenting its effect on fracture rates haven't been done; therefore, ERT is FDA-approved only for prevention and not for the treatment of osteoporosis. Estrogen's benefits are not reduced when a progestogen is added (known as hormone replacement therapy or HRT) for women with a uterus.

Pros: Many ERT and HRT products have been proven effective and are FDA-approved for preventing postmenopausal bone loss. ERT/HRT provides other potential benefits, such as reducing hot flashes, insomnia, and vaginal dryness, and it may be helpful in lowering the risk of heart disease. **Cons**: ERT must be used long-term because when therapy stops, significant bone loss resumes. Some women on long-term ERT may continue to experience bone loss, and it may be necessary to measure bone density periodically. ERT can increase uterine cancer risk, but adding a progestogen reduces that risk to, or possibly even below, the level of taking no hormones at all. Long-term use of ERT/HRT may increase the risk of breast cancer. Estrogen should not be used in women with a history of blood clots or during periods of prolonged immobilization (see ERT; Progestogen & HRT).

A BMD measurement at menopause may be helpful in making an informed decision about osteoporosis treatment.

Bisphosphonates. These are nonhormonal, bone-specific drugs that decrease the activity of bone-dissolving cells. **Pros**: These drugs preserve bone density and bone strength as well as reduce fracture risk. **Cons**: Because food reduces their absorption, bisphosphonates must be taken on an empty stomach, with water only, and at least 30 minutes before drinking other liquids, eating, or taking other medicines. Bisphosphonates in general use are alendronate, risedronate, and etidronate.

- **Alendronate** (Fosamax tablets) is approved in the United States and Canada for post-menopausal osteoporosis prevention and treatment. It significantly increases bone density in the spine and hip and decreases the risk of spine and nonspine fractures. Alendronate is available in both a daily and a once-weekly dose.

- **Risedronate** (Actonel tablets) is also approved for postmenopausal osteoporosis prevention and treatment. It is similar to alendronate in its effect on bone density and fracture reduction. Risedronate has been shown to significantly reduce hip fractures in women with osteoporosis. It also reduces the risk of spine fractures after only one year of therapy. Risedronate requires daily dosing.

- **Etidronate** (Didronel tablets) is FDA-approved for the treatment of another bone disorder, Paget's disease. Nevertheless, some clinicians prescribe it in lower doses for postmenopausal osteoporosis. In Canada, it is approved for osteoporosis treatment, and it is also available in combination with calcium (Didrocal). When prescribed for osteoporosis, it must be taken cyclically (eg, two weeks out of every three months, then repeated) to prevent abnormalities in bone mineralization.

Calcitonin. This drug is marketed as Calcimar injections or Miacalcin injections or nasal spray. Calcitonin is a hormone, but not a steroid hormone, such as estrogen. It is approved in the United States and Canada for the treatment (not the prevention) of osteoporosis. **Pros:** It results in slight gains in spine bone density, but the increase is less than that seen with estrogen or bisphosphonates. Calcitonin also significantly decreases spine fractures, and it may reduce pain from spinal fractures. It is relatively safe and has no serious side effects. **Cons:** Minor nose irritation has been observed with the nasal spray. It has not been shown to prevent nonspine fractures. Calcitonin is less potent than the other options, and it is recommended only for women who are five years beyond menopause because efficacy has not been observed in the early postmenopausal years.

Raloxifene. This drug, marketed as Evista tablets, is approved in the United States and Canada for the prevention and treatment of osteoporosis. Raloxifene is in a class of drugs called SERMs (selective estrogen receptor modulators), which act like estrogen in some parts of the body. **Pros:** Raloxifene increases bone density, although to a lesser degree than estrogen or alendronate. It does not appear to harm the breast or uterus. Ongoing research may reveal beneficial actions beyond bone. **Cons:** Unlike estrogen, raloxifene does not help with short-term menopause symptoms, such as hot flashes, and actually causes hot flashes in some women. Like estrogen, it cannot be used in women with a history of blood clots or during periods of prolonged immobilization.

Other agents. Several agents are sometimes prescribed by clinicians for treating bone loss, but none is FDA-approved for this use. Phytoestrogens offer promise, but more research is needed (see Complementary & Alternative Medicines). New therapies are being studied and may be approved in the near future, including parathyroid hormone and tibolone.

CANCER

Menopause is not associated with an increased risk of cancer. However, since cancer rates typically increase with age, women must be aware of the most common cancers that affect women. Also, some of the therapies used for menopause are associated with an increase or a decrease in the incidence of certain types of cancer.

Each year, thousands of women are cured of cancer, and those diagnosed today have a much better chance of living longer than in the past. In North America, about two out of every five women diagnosed with cancer will be alive five years after diagnosis. Even more women are reducing their risk by learning to be "cancer smart." Being informed and discussing concerns with a healthcare provider are key steps toward optimal health. The most common types of cancer for women are presented in the following sections.

Breast Cancer

Breast cancer is perhaps the cancer women fear most. This fear comes from the possibility of dying from the disease, but also from the rigorous demands of treatment and the probability of cancer recurrence. Many midlife women have personally seen relatives or friends go through breast cancer treatment or have lost loved ones to the disease.

Breast cancer is the second major cause of cancer death in North American women. Fortunately, the death rate has started to decline in recent years. Smaller, less-advanced cancers can now be detected earlier with mammography.

US statistics show that if breast cancer is detected while still localized, the five-year survival rate is 96% – a dramatic improvement from 72% in the 1940s. The same improvements in cancer survival have also been seen in Canadian women. Several factors have been identified as increasing the risk of breast cancer (see box below).

Role of ERT/HRT. There is controversy about a possible relationship and the magnitude of any relationship between the development of breast cancer and estrogen replacement therapy (ERT) or, for women with a uterus, combined estrogen plus progestogen therapy (hormone replacement therapy or HRT). ERT/HRT probably does not cause breast cancer, but it may stimulate cancer cells to grow. Studies conducted in the 1990s to determine a more precise relationship between ERT/HRT and breast cancer produced conflicting results. Most experts believe that the incidence of breast cancer is not affected by short-term ERT/HRT use (5 to 10 years or less), but may increase with longer therapy. The Women's Health Initiative, a large national study, may provide more definitive answers when the study concludes in 2005. However, many experts believe that additional studies will only confirm the variability and inconsistency of the findings to date and that no study can be designed so that a clear conclusion can be reached.

Menopause is not associated with increased cancer risks.

Factors That Increase Breast Cancer Risk

Age: A woman's risk of breast cancer increases with age. Nearly half of all cases occur in women 65 years and older. Current estimates predict that by age 50, 2% of US and Canadian women will have developed breast cancer – by 60, about 5%; by 70, about 7%; and by 80, about 10%.

Genetics: A woman's risk of developing breast cancer is also increased if her mother or sister had the disease, especially if before menopause. However, since most breast cancers occur in women without a positive family history, every woman needs to be concerned.

Menstrual periods beginning before 12 years of age.

Never having children.

Having a first child after age 30.

Being obese or more than 20% over ideal weight.

Drinking alcohol; two to five drinks daily increases risk by about 40%.

Lack of exercise.

Diet low in vegetables and fruit.

Radiation treatment for other cancers.

Other factors such as high-fat diet and exposure to certain pesticides.

Long-term ERT/HRT.

Many women use ERT/HRT for relief of hot flashes, for which there is no other comparable effective treatment. They usually have prompt relief and can taper off hormones long before excess breast cancer risk is evident. The decision to continue hormones over the long term, as necessary to prevent osteoporosis, is more complicated. Here, it is especially important for each woman to weigh her individual risks and benefits. No simple rule will apply to every woman, as each has her own risks and concerns.

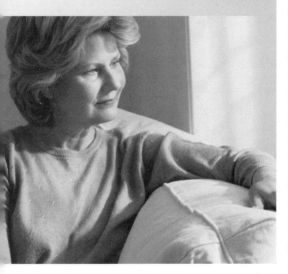

Since many breast cancer risk factors cannot be changed, early detection is the best strategy for optimal outcomes.

Having a history of or a high-risk profile for breast cancer is not considered to be an absolute contraindication for ERT/HRT use. In certain situations, the clinician — in consultation with the woman's oncologist — may help the woman decide whether the benefits of such therapy appear to outweigh its risks. The decision must be made with the full awareness that therapy might promote more rapid tumor growth.

For women who cannot or choose not to use long-term ERT/HRT to prevent osteoporosis due to their risk profile for breast cancer, the SERM raloxifene (see Osteoporosis) offers an attractive alternative, as some studies suggest that raloxifene may not only be safe for the breast, but may even help prevent breast cancer. Another SERM, tamoxifen (Nolvadex), is FDA-approved to treat breast cancer. Short-term use (less than five years) has been shown to reduce the risk of breast cancer in women at high risk; however, tamoxifen is not considered effective for osteoporosis. Both raloxifene and tamoxifen are associated with an increase in hot flashes, whereas tamoxifen is associated with an increased risk of uterine cancer. Like estrogen, both SERMs are associated with an increased risk for blood clots in the legs and lungs.

Early detection. Since many breast cancer risk factors cannot be altered, early detection is the best strategy for optimal health. Once a woman reaches adulthood, it is recommended that she self-examine her breasts monthly and have them examined by a healthcare provider during an annual physical check-up. The best time for both a manual exam and a mammogram (breast x-ray) is immediately after monthly menstrual bleeding stops (if menstruating) or after bleeding caused by some types of HRT stops (see Progestogen & HRT) because breasts are less dense then.

If anything unusual is found, such as a lump or nipple discharge, both a mammogram and clinical follow-up are appropriate. Recommendations for mammography screening vary. In the absence of unusual findings, NAMS recommends annual mammograms beginning at age 40 and continuing throughout life. NAMS also recommends a mammogram before initiating ERT/HRT. The value of mammograms in premenopausal women is controversial, because they are harder to read and have more false positives. Women with fibrocystic (lumpy) breasts or breast implants will have more dense breasts, making abnormalities more difficult to detect. ERT/HRT use also makes breasts appear more dense.

Ultrasound is becoming more popular as a means to investigate suspicious mammogram findings.

Although most breast lumps are noncancerous, all lumps should be evaluated. A biopsy may be necessary to rule out cancer. Studies repeatedly show that early diagnosis is linked to higher cure rates.

Endometrial (Uterine) Cancer

Cancer can affect the inside lining of the uterus, called the endometrium. Fewer than 3 in 100 women past age 50 will develop endometrial cancer in their remaining lifetime, and far fewer will die from the disease. When detected early, endometrial cancer has a five-year survival rate of 95%.

Risk factors for developing endometrial cancer include use of estrogen without progestogen, use of tamoxifen, early menarche (starting periods early), reaching menopause late, missing periods during menstruating years (not including pregnancy), infertility or never being pregnant, obesity, diabetes, high blood pressure, gallbladder disease, and, perhaps, hereditary colon cancer. Previous pregnancy and oral contraceptive use appear to provide some protection against endometrial cancer. Annual pelvic exams are recommended for all peri- and postmenopausal women. For high-risk women, the American Cancer Society also recommends an endometrial biopsy once menopause is reached. Abnormal uterine bleeding is one of the first signs of endometrial cancer. If noted, an endometrial biopsy will probably be required. The Pap test, which is so effective in detecting cervical cancer, is not a reliable test to detect uterine cancer. Since the thickness of the endometrium may provide clues, transvaginal ultrasound and sonohysterography (viewing the uterus filled with salt water) are being used by some clinicians to look for endometrial cancer and other causes of postmenopausal bleeding.

Role of ERT/HRT. Using ERT without a progestogen, also called "unopposed ERT," over a period of three or more years has been associated with a marked increase in endometrial cancer.

Most endometrial cancers that appear while taking unopposed ERT are low-grade cancers and do not reduce a woman's lifespan if detected early and cured with a hysterectomy. Using the proper type and amount of progestogen with ERT counteracts the increased risk of endometrial cancer, reducing the risk to, or possibly even below, the level of taking no hormones at all. Thus, all women with an intact uterus should use a progestogen with ERT (see Progestogen & HRT).

Cervical Cancer

The death rate from cervical cancer has dropped sharply in the United States and Canada, but it remains a serious concern. Today, 25% of all new cases and more than 40% of all deaths from cervical cancer occur in US women over age 60. In Canada, about 29% of all new cases occur in women over age 60, and 64% of all deaths occur in women over age 55. The incidence rate is about 11 per 100,000 in black women and around 7 per 100,000 in white women. If diagnosed early, cervical cancer is highly treatable; its five-year survival rate is 91%.

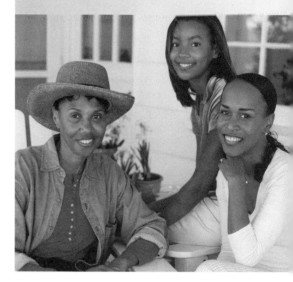

A Pap test reliably detects cervical cancer, but it cannot be relied on to detect cancer of the uterus.

Cervical cancer is now understood to be caused by the human papillomavirus (HPV), an infection acquired primarily through sexual relations. Most HPV infections, however, do not lead to cancer. Neither menopause nor ERT/HRT use has been linked to increased cervical cancer risk. The likelihood for HPV infection increases with the following: sexual intercourse at an early age, multiple sexual partners, sexual partners who have had multiple partners, smoking, and HIV infection. In both men and women, HPV infection is sometimes associated with benign (noncancerous) growths in the genital area, called genital warts (condyloma). Most women have no signs or symptoms of HPV even though they carry the virus. Spread of HPV may be reduced considerably by the use of condoms.

The Pap smear is a screening test for any abnormal change in the cells of the cervix. Having a regular Pap smear test will usually allow for the early discovery of these abnormal changes. This also determines whether a woman needs a closer look at the cervix through an instrument called a colposcope. Despite the importance of the Pap test, about 50% of US women diagnosed with cervical cancer have never had one. The Pap test is a simple office procedure in which cells are swabbed from the cervix and analyzed under a microscope. Properly performed, the test can detect abnormal cells before they become cancerous.

Regular Pap tests are needed throughout a woman's life.

For all peri- and postmenopausal women, NAMS recommends a pelvic exam every year and a Pap test every three years, unless an abnormality is detected. An annual Pap test is important for women at high risk, including those who are not in a mutually monogamous, steady relationship; those who have had genital warts or have HIV infection (or AIDS); or those who are current or past smokers.

If a Pap test shows abnormalities or if there is a history of cancer, testing may be needed more often than yearly. Although the Pap test evaluates the cervix (opening to uterus), even after hysterectomy (in which the cervix is typically removed along with the uterus), a Pap test may be recommended to detect precancers in the vagina and in any remaining cervical tissues.

Ovarian Cancer

Statistics show that American and Canadian women have a low incidence of cancer of the ovaries. Ovarian cancer represents about 4% of all cancers, yet it causes more deaths than any other cancer of the reproductive system, primarily because it usually appears in an advanced and less curable stage. When ovarian cancer is detected early, 95% of women survive at least five years.

Neither menopause nor ERT/HRT use has been linked to ovarian cancer. Risk for ovarian cancer increases with age, particularly in women without children or those with a family history of breast or ovarian cancer. Lowered risk of ovarian cancer is associated with previous pregnancy, past use of birth control pills, and having a bilateral tubal ligation (tubes "tied" to prevent pregnancy).

Because there are no satisfactory screening tests available for ovarian cancer, an annual pelvic exam is recommended, especially for women over age 40. Pap tests rarely discover ovarian cancer. Transvaginal ultrasound and a blood test for the tumor marker CA125 have been used for screening women at high risk for ovarian cancer, but studies have not proven the value of this approach.

Recent research suggests a potential link between the use of genital talcum powder and ovarian cancer. Thus, the use of talcum powder between the legs is not recommended.

Lung Cancer

Today, lung cancer is the leading cause of cancer death in North American women, surpassing the long-time leader, breast cancer. The number of newly diagnosed cases continues to rise. These alarming statistics parallel the increasing numbers of women who smoke cigarettes, by far the most important risk factor in developing this disease.

Of all the lifestyle-related risk factors that can be changed, smoking cessation has the greatest impact on reducing death rates, not only from lung cancer but also from other serious diseases, including an increased risk of cervical cancer. Nonsmokers' exposure to second-hand tobacco smoke also poses health risks. One study reports that the risk of lung cancer is approximately 30% higher for wives of smokers than for wives of nonsmokers.

Colon & Rectal Cancer

After lung and breast cancer, colorectal cancer is the next most common cause of cancer death in US women. This includes cancers of the colon (the lower part of the intestine) and the rectum (the part of the intestine that leads from the colon to the anus). Colorectal cancer is not associated with menopause but with age; colorectal cancer incidence is six times higher in women aged 65 years and older compared with women aged 40 to 64 years. Other factors that increase the risk include a family history of colorectal cancer, colorectal polyps, inflammatory bowel disease, physical inactivity, low calcium intake, low folate intake, and smoking.

Colorectal cancer risk may be lowered through exercise, healthy eating habits, high calcium intake (1,200 mg/day), and estrogen replacement therapy.

Colon cancer begins as precancerous colon polyps. It can be prevented if the polyps are detected and removed before they become cancerous. When colorectal cancer is found early, 90% of those treated will survive at least five years.

For women at average risk for colorectal cancer, NAMS recommends an annual rectal exam and test of stool for blood (called a fecal occult blood test) after age 50, and flexible sigmoidoscopy (a test to view inside the rectum and lower colon) every three to five years after age 50. Colonoscopy is recommended to view areas beyond the reach of the sigmoidoscope, especially in women at high risk.

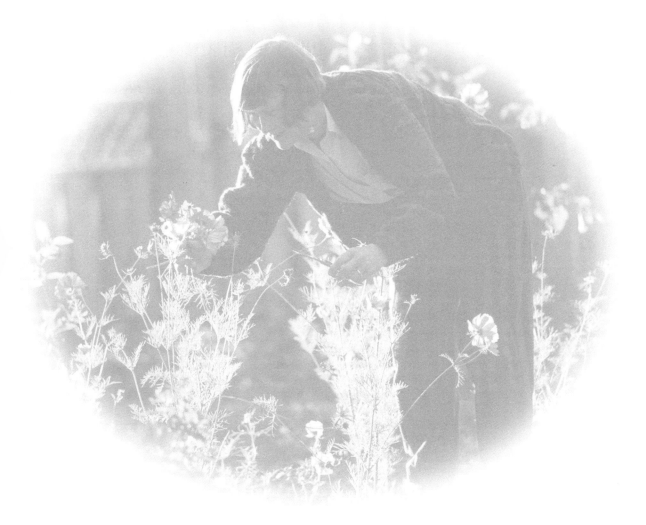

MENOPAUSE TREATMENT OPTIONS

TO MAKE INFORMED HEALTH DECISIONS

APPROPRIATE FOR INDIVIDUAL LIFE

SITUATIONS, WOMEN NEED INFORMATION

ON AVAILABLE TREATMENT OPTIONS TO

EASE THE MENOPAUSAL TRANSITION AND

REDUCE RISK OF DISEASE LATER IN LIFE.

THEY ALSO NEED A HEALTHCARE PROVIDER

THEY CAN TRUST TO HAVE AN OPEN

DISCUSSION OF THEIR HEALTH CONCERNS.

A CLINICIAN WITH EXPERTISE IN

MANAGING MENOPAUSE CAN OFFER

OPTIMAL CARE, ESPECIALLY FOR WOMEN

WITH TROUBLESOME SYMPTOMS OR

COMPLEX RISK PROFILES.

Some health changes associated with menopause – such as hot flashes, mood swings, irregular bleeding, and difficulty sleeping – are acute (short-term) effects, typically lasting a few months or a few years during perimenopause and early postmenopause. They will usually go away on their own, even without treatment. Prolonged periods of reduced estrogen levels, however, have the potential to cause chronic (long-term) effects in later years, such as osteoporosis, vaginal atrophy, and, possibly, heart disease.

A full discussion with a healthcare provider about present disturbances and future health risks will help determine an individual woman's best treatment options. Some women will find treatment improves their quality of life significantly. Other women do not require or request specific medical management for the hormonal changes of menopause and choose only to maintain a healthy lifestyle. However, all women will benefit from a visit to their healthcare provider to make sure that the decisions they are making about their health are informed decisions.

For acute symptoms of menopause and for lowering the risk of chronic diseases that can increase after menopause, various treatment options are available, including lifestyle changes, nonprescription remedies, prescription therapies, and complementary and alternative medicine (CAM) therapies. These four categories of options are discussed fully in the next sections of this booklet.

LIFESTYLE CHANGES

Positive lifestyle changes can have an enormous impact on health. A customized lifestyle modification strategy is an essential element in a comprehensive therapeutic plan that can apply to a woman throughout her life span. These adjustable lifestyle choices include substance use, exercise, nutrition, weight management, and stress reduction.

Substance Use

Use of tobacco and illegal substances, as well as excessive use of alcohol and caffeine, contribute to poor health. Without doubt, smoking is the single most preventable cause of illness and premature death. The reasons to quit or never to start are numerous. Smoking increases the risk of heart and lung disease, osteoporosis, and many types of cancer, including lung and cervical cancer. It may double the risk of Alzheimer's disease and other similar mental diseases. Smokers may also experience menopause up to two years earlier than nonsmokers.

Smoking is the single greatest preventable cause of illness and premature death.

Many women successfully quit smoking, sometimes after several attempts. Healthcare providers can offer a variety of smoking cessation aids, including prescription nicotine products (in gum or skin patch regimens) and antidepressants to decrease psychological dependence on smoking. Nicotine products and one antidepressant (Zyban) are FDA-approved to help "kick the habit." Support groups and hypnosis are other potentially helpful options. A combination of behavior modification techniques and prescription drug therapy appears to be the most successful.

Adequate Exercise

For many serious diseases, physical inactivity is a lifestyle risk factor. Adequate exercise is a crucial ingredient often missing from daily life. Brisk walking, running, aerobics, dancing, tennis, and weight-training are but a few of the activities that help the heart, bones, muscles, balance, and body weight.

Proper exercise is a powerful remedy for many menopause complaints and can help prevent future menopause-related diseases. It promotes better, more restorative sleep, and it stimulates production of "feel-good" brain chemistry (endorphins) that turns aside negative thoughts and depressed feelings. Some women report having fewer hot flashes when they exercise regularly. A key first step is to develop a practical, long-term, individually suited exercise plan.

There are three types of exercise: aerobic, weight-bearing, and flexibility (stretching). A moderate aerobic exercise regimen of at least 30 minutes each day has the greatest effect on heart and lung health. A brisk two-mile walk is a good aerobic exercise. Weight-bearing exercise, such as walking or working with weights to build muscle, can delay or prevent bone loss. Early in life, exercise promotes higher bone mass; later in life, it can have a modest effect on declining bone loss. Flexibility exercises, such as yoga and stretching, help maintain function while aging and may improve balance, which can decrease the risk of fractures caused by falls.

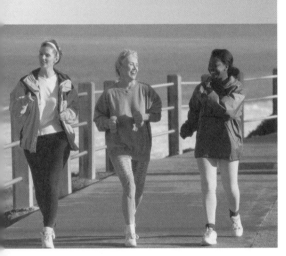

Exercise is a powerful remedy for many menopause complaints.

A healthcare provider can help determine the initial level of exercise appropriate for individual needs. Then, finding ways to make exercise a permanent part of daily life will help ensure a healthier future.

Healthy Diet

"You are what you eat" may sound trite, but it's true. A balanced diet low in saturated fat and high in whole grains, fruits, and vegetables, with adequate water, vitamins, and minerals contributes to good health. Women at perimenopause and beyond have special dietary concerns, because both heart disease and osteoporosis are greatly affected by diet.

Heart disease risk can be lowered by using little or no cholesterol or animal fat. Instead, choose olive or canola oil for cooking, and avoid hydrogenated oil found in some peanut butters and margarines. Limit salt and alcohol intake, include five or more servings daily of fruits and vegetables, and include soy foods (such as soy milk and tofu) to lower cholesterol levels (see Phytoestrogens & Soy).

A balanced diet is important for bone development and maintaining bone strength. Some women – especially those who are elderly and have reduced appetites, who diet frequently, who don't consume dairy products, or who have eating disorders – may not consume adequate vitamins and minerals to maintain optimal bone mass.

Osteoporosis risk can be lowered by an adequate intake of calcium, starting in the teen years. This builds bone mass and bone strength to a peak during the 20s and allows the body to draw from this "bone bank account" from then on. As women reach menopause, consuming adequate calcium is still important as ever. NAMS recommends that postmenopausal women consume 1,200 to 1,500 mg of elemental calcium daily. This is significantly more than the average amount consumed each day by women aged 50 to 65 (only 700 mg).

Calcium intake can be increased by eating more calcium-rich dairy products (low-fat or nonfat preferred). A glass of milk or portion of other dairy product provides about 300 mg of calcium. Increased intake of leafy green vegetables and calcium-fortified foods and juices also increases calcium intake. If sufficient calcium is not found in the diet, a calcium supplement can be used (see Nonprescription Remedies).

Vitamin D also plays a major role in helping the body absorb calcium. At least 15 minutes of sun exposure daily (without a sunscreen) is the generally accepted amount the body needs to form its supply. Certain foods (such as fortified milk, liver, and tuna) or a vitamin D supplement can help reach the recommended daily level for postmenopausal women – 400 to 600 IU (see Nonprescription Remedies).

New research suggests that at least this amount is needed by women who are never in the sun or who live in northern regions.

Weight Management

Being overweight increases the risk of heart disease and invites other diseases, such as diabetes and arthritis. The most dangerous location of body fat for heart health is the waistline and stomach. As they age, midlife women often gain two pounds a year. When diet and exercise are not enough to control weight, support groups or weight-management organizations may help. Additional therapies are available for those who have a more severe weight problem.

Being too thin is not necessarily healthy either. Premenopausal women who over-diet or over-exercise can become so thin that their menstrual periods stop temporarily. This temporary low estrogen state increases the risk of osteoporosis later in life. Everyone needs to work on strategies to maintain a healthy weight.

Stress Reduction

Prolonged stress can have a severe impact on health. Although menopause has not been shown to raise stress levels, women at midlife face many stressors, some of them new. A number of coping strategies can be used to help reduce stress (see Psychological Changes). Exercise and meditation may help. Deep, slow, abdominal breathing can increase relaxation and may also reduce hot flashes. Some women report fewer hot flashes when they engage in meditation, yoga, massage, or just a leisurely bath. It is beneficial to reduce stress and take time to relax each day. Women need to care for themselves, both physically and spiritually.

NONPRESCRIPTION REMEDIES

There are many products available without a prescription ("over-the-counter") that may help with specific menopause-related complaints. Healthcare professionals can provide information about these products, including vitamin and mineral supplements, other nutritional supplements, and vaginal lubricants and moisturizers. A woman's healthcare provider should be involved in the decision to use nonprescription products because no therapy is without potential risk.

Vitamins & Minerals

Probably every woman could benefit from a good quality, daily multivitamin and mineral supplement.

After menopause, the chosen supplement typically should not contain iron, because a woman no longer loses iron through menstrual bleeding. During perimenopause, when periods may be quite heavy, the clinician may recommend that a woman take extra iron to avoid anemia.

Most daily supplements contain 400 IU of vitamin D, providing the amount that most women need. For those who are never in the sun, 600 IU is recommended.

A woman's healthcare provider should be involved in the decision to use any product available without a prescription because no therapy is without potential risk.

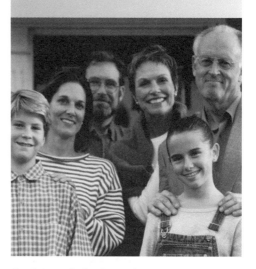

A "multi" preparation may not contain the daily requirement of calcium, however, because the tablet would be too large. If adequate calcium cannot be obtained from the diet, a separate calcium supplement may be required to reach the recommended level of 1,200 to 1,500 mg elemental calcium daily. Several types of calcium are available, such as calcium carbonate (eg, Tums) and calcium citrate (eg, Citracal). Calcium-fortified foods provide another source.

Regulations For Dietary Supplements

In early 2000, the FDA began allowing dietary supplement marketers to make health claims for certain conditions without providing documentation for efficacy or safety. These conditions include hot flashes and age-related memory loss, for example, but not prevention of diseases, such as osteoporosis and heart disease. The marketer, not the FDA, is responsible for ensuring that labels are truthful and not misleading, that they contain enough information for consumers to make an informed choice, and that all dietary ingredients are accurately listed.

Some women choose a combination supplement of calcium and vitamin D (eg, Oscal). Calcium is best absorbed when taken with meals in 250 to 500 mg doses throughout the day. Calcium should not be taken with fiber or iron supplements. Up to 1,500 mg of calcium per day does not increase the risk of kidney stones, but drinking plenty of water is advised.

Some women find vitamin E (daily doses of 400 IU or more) helpful in reducing hot flashes, although studies do not support this benefit. For easiest digestion, this supplement should be taken along with a meal that contains fats. It may take two to six weeks before feeling the optimum effects, if any. Vitamin E supplements thin the blood, so these supplements should not be used by women using blood-thinning prescription drugs or aspirin.

Other vitamins and minerals are available over-the-counter. A woman's healthcare provider can provide guidance regarding her needs for these products.

Hormones

Also available without a prescription are products containing hormones such as topical progesterone and DHEA, marketed under the dietary supplement regulations (see box). None of these products is FDA-approved to treat a menopause-related condition.

Topical progesterone creams. These come in strengths ranging from 2 to 400 mg per ounce and are marketed for a variety of claims, including relief of hot flashes and protection against osteoporosis and breast cancer. These claims have not been confirmed through clinical studies.

Studies with one topical progesterone cream have shown that after applying the cream on the skin's surface, progesterone is absorbed into the bloodstream, but studies show that the products are not consistent in delivering levels high enough to protect the uterus when using estrogen replacement therapy. Some topical progesterone products have been found to contain no progesterone at all. A prescription progestogen is a better choice to provide the needed protection. Because of these concerns, NAMS does not recommend the use of over-the-counter progesterone creams.

DHEA (dehydroepiandrosterone) is an androgen hormone made by the human adrenal gland. It can be synthesized from wild yams. DHEA is marketed with a wide range of claims, such as improving immune function, slowing the aging process, increasing energy, improving cholesterol levels, causing weight loss, improving mood, and increasing sex drive.

However, very few clinical trials have been conducted regarding its use in humans, and more are needed to support not only its effectiveness but also its safety. Because of these reasons, NAMS does not recommend its use. High doses can produce side effects, such as liver damage and depressed mood. DHEA is contraindicated in women who have a history of hormone-sensitive tumors or who might become pregnant (because of possible masculinization of a female fetus).

Vaginal Lubricants & Moisturizers

Minor vaginal moisture problems can often be solved by using one of many water-soluble vaginal products designed for this use. A wide selection of lubricants (eg, Astroglide, Lubrin, Moist Again) and moisturizers (eg, Replens, K-Y Long-Lasting) are available. Unlike lubricants, moisturizers act directly on tissue to make it less dry. Moisturizers have the extra advantage of a low pH that helps keep the vagina acidic and less inviting for infection.

Only products designed for vaginal dryness are recommended. Hand lotion contains ingredients such as alcohol and perfume that can irritate vaginal tissue. Oil-based products such as Vaseline petroleum jelly and baby oil can also cause irritation, damage condoms and diaphragms, and cling to vaginal tissue, providing a habitat for infection. One exception may be vitamin E oil, which some women have found to provide lubrication and relieve itching and irritation.

Vinegar douches and vaginally applied cultures of lactobacilli or yogurt are not effective for vaginal dryness and are not recommended. Antihistamine pills taken for allergies have a drying effect on all mucous membranes, including those in the nose and in the vaginal wall. It is also advisable to limit the use of soap, bubble baths, and bath oils as well as to avoid talcum powder in the vaginal area because of a possible link with ovarian cancer.

No vaginal lubricant or moisturizer treats the cause of menopause-related vaginal dryness and atrophy. Since the cause is a lack of estrogen, vaginal tissue can best be restored with prescription estrogen therapy. Estrogen is FDA-approved for treating vaginal atrophy.

PRESCRIPTION THERAPIES

Several prescription drugs are available to help with menopause-related changes. By far, the most often used drug for these conditions is the hormone estrogen, which is prescribed to replace the lowered levels secreted by the ovaries at menopause. Estrogen is FDA-approved for the treatment of hot flashes and vaginal atrophy as well as the prevention of osteoporosis. A number of factors need to be considered when a woman, with the guidance of her healthcare provider, decides whether therapy with estrogen is right for her. There is no "one size fits all" when it comes to menopause therapy. Each woman is unique and must make her own decision after totally understanding her personal situation.

ERT

Therapy with estrogen for menopause-related conditions is usually called estrogen replacement therapy (ERT). However, the term "replacement" is a misnomer because ERT provides only a small fraction of the estrogen once produced by the ovaries; estrogen supplementation is more accurate. ERT has been widely studied and used for more than 50 years by millions of women. ERT is unique because it has the potential to help with a wide range of short-term disturbances, such as hot flashes and vaginal dryness. It also has the potential to prevent major diseases, such as osteoporosis and, possibly, heart disease. Some women report that they simply "feel good" while on therapy. Thus, if a woman needs therapy for many conditions, ERT can be viewed as relatively economical "one stop shopping." If fewer conditions need treatment or if ERT is not an option, more targeted therapies must be used, usually one therapy for each condition. There are

> *ERT stands for Estrogen Replacement Therapy.*
>
> *HRT stands for Hormone Replacement Therapy, a combination of estrogen plus progestogen to protect the uterus.*

many approaches other than ERT for treating acute disturbances and preventing major diseases related to menopause.

Estrogen benefits women at particular risk for osteoporosis. Its role in prevention of heart disease, Alzheimer's disease, and other conditions later in life is still unclear. Women who have no identifiable risk factors for these diseases may still benefit from estrogen use for treatment of short-term conditions. Research is currently underway to determine which women will benefit most from estrogen therapy, at what dosage, and at what time of life.

Dosage forms of ERT. Several dosage forms of ERT are available, allowing a woman who needs estrogen to use exactly what is best for her:

- **Systemic.** When administered as an oral tablet, skin patch, intravenous injection, or in a custom-made product such as a pellet implanted under the skin, estrogen circulates throughout the body's system (hence the term "systemic"), affecting many different tissues. All of these forms have the potential to reduce or completely stop the short-term disturbances of menopause and help in preventing osteoporosis and, possibly, heart disease. Although available, estrogen injections are not recommended for menopause therapy, since the estrogen level in the blood tends to peak too high after an injection and goes too low between injections, causing adverse effects.

- **Local.** When administered as a vaginal cream, vaginal ring, or vaginal tablet, estrogen is considered "local" therapy (one that affects only a specific or localized area of the body). Local dosage forms of ERT are available to treat vaginal dryness and more severe vaginal atrophy and are, therefore, sometimes called "vaginal" forms. With a local form, only a very small amount of estrogen circulates through the body. Therefore, vaginal ERT rarely helps with hot flashes or the prevention

Estrogen Products FDA-Approved For Postmenopausal Use

ESTROGEN TYPE	ORAL TABLET PRODUCT NAME	SKIN PATCH PRODUCT NAME	VAGINAL FORM PRODUCT NAME
conjugated equine estrogens	Premarin	Not available	Premarin Vaginal Cream
synthetic conjugated estrogens	Cenestin	Not available	Not available
esterified estrogens	Estratab, Menest	Not available	Not available
estropipate (piperazine estrone sulfate)	Ortho-Est, Ogen	Not available	Ogen Vaginal Cream
micronized 17-beta-estradiol	Estrace	**Matrix patch:** Alora, Climara, Esclim, Vivelle, Vivelle-Dot **Reservoir patch:** Estraderm	Estrace Vaginal Cream, Estring Vaginal Ring
estradiol hemihydrate	Not available	Not available	Vagifem Vaginal Tablet

of osteoporosis and heart disease. However, enough estrogen may get into the blood to possibly affect the uterus, so progestogen therapy is sometimes prescribed along with vaginal ERT (especially with the cream form) to protect the uterus.

ERT types. In addition to various dosage forms, various types of estrogen are available in many products FDA-approved for postmenopausal use (see box). No ERT is approved for use before menopause, although many clinicians offer ERT for relief of symptoms during this transition time, and it frequently works.

Custom-made formulations are prepared by a compounding pharmacist from a prescription. They allow even more specific tailoring of therapy, depending on what's best for a particular woman. Often-prescribed custom estrogen products are estriol cream and Tri-Est (a mixture of three estrogens: 80% estriol, 10% estrone, and 10% 17-beta-estradiol). Most women do not need customized formulations. Although much may be known about the active estrogen ingredient(s), little or nothing is known about the custom formulation that delivers the estrogen into the body. While the active ingredient is FDA-approved, the formulation is not. These products have not been tested in proper scientific studies as to purity, reliability, effectiveness, safety, and optimal dose. Since custom products are experimental, they must be used with caution.

The availability of estrogen in a variety of dosage forms, types, and strengths gives each woman a better chance to find what is best for her. Finding the right regimen may require time, patience, and trying various prescriptions and delivery systems.

Women who should not use ERT. Some women have risk factors that are contraindications to ERT use. Contraindications are reasons not to use treatment. However, the potential benefits sometimes outweigh the potential risks, leading a few women to accept therapy after careful consideration. In general, women who have the following should not use ERT:

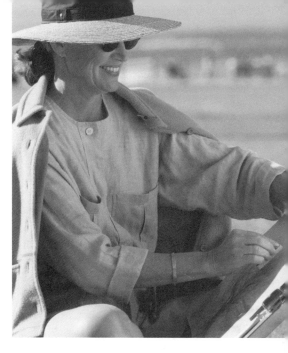

- Known or suspected pregnancy;

- History of breast cancer;

- History of hormone-sensitive cancer;

- Unexplained uterine bleeding;

- History of blood-clotting disorders.

Cigarette smoking is not a contraindication for ERT, as it is with oral contraceptive use in older women, but smokers are urged to stop before treatment starts for general health reasons.

Side effects of ERT. Potential side effects of ERT are listed below. Many of these side effects can be managed using a variety of techniques (see Dealing with ERT/HRT Side Effects on page 49).

- Uterine bleeding (starting or returning);

- Breast tenderness (sometimes enlargement);

- Nausea;

- Abdominal bloating;

- Fluid retention in extremities;

- Changes in the shape of the cornea of the eye (sometimes leading to contact lens intolerance);

- Headache (sometimes migraine);

- Dizziness;

- Increased breast density (making mammograms more difficult to interpret).

Estrogen does not cause weight gain. However, in some women, ERT can cause fluid retention in the hands and feet and/or abdominal bloating with gaseous bowel distension, sometimes resulting in a temporary weight gain. Increasing fluid intake, limiting salt consumption and participating in regular exercise will help reduce water retention.

There is one "side effect" issue that is important to keep in mind when ERT is to be discontinued — stopping all at once typically brings on hot flashes. Tapering the dose over time is advised.

ERT and cancer risk concerns. Estrogen probably does not cause cancer, but it may cause estrogen-

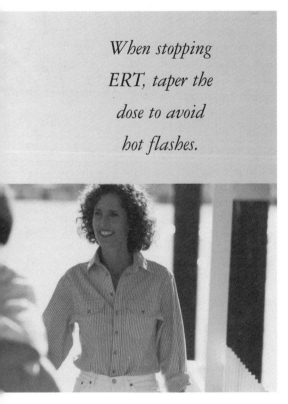

When stopping ERT, taper the dose to avoid hot flashes.

sensitive cancer cells to grow. It is well documented that using estrogen for five or more years can triple the risk of developing cancer of the endometrium. However, it is also well known that adding another prescription hormone – progestogen – to estrogen therapy reduces that risk to, or possibly even below, the level of taking no hormones. Combined estrogen and progestogen therapy is known as hormone replacement therapy or HRT (see Endometrial Cancer; Progestogen & HRT).

Many women reject estrogen because they fear it may increase their risk of breast cancer. The relationship between hormones and breast cancer is currently a controversial issue (see Breast Cancer). There is no evidence that the dosage known to relieve hot flashes and other acute changes during perimenopause increases the risk of breast cancer in the short term. However, the risk increases by as much as 40% when estrogen is used for long periods of time (defined by some studies as five years or more).

Thus, there is concern regarding ERT/HRT use for many years to help prevent diseases, such as

osteoporosis, that may not strike for 15 or more years after menopause.

Some scientists point out that the risk of breast or uterine cancer with ERT/HRT use is small compared with the benefits, which include the possibility of reducing the risk of heart disease. Heart disease is the leading cause of death for women. In fact, the risk of death from heart disease is many times higher than from breast cancer. In the United States, for example, a female at birth has a 23% lifetime risk of dying from heart disease compared with a 4% risk of breast cancer and 2.5% risk of bone fractures from osteoporosis. Further research will hopefully clarify some of the current uncertainties.

Weighing benefits and risks of ERT. Studies have conclusively documented that estrogen taken for many years helps prevent osteoporosis and may also decrease the risk of heart disease. However, estrogen's protection against these diseases depends on its long-term, continuous use, which may increase a woman's risk of breast cancer. Each woman must decide for herself if these potential rewards outweigh the potential risk. Only after examining and understanding her own situation and after a thorough consultation with her healthcare provider can a woman make the best treatment choice.

An informed decision does not rely on impersonal statistics or someone else's choice. It relies on the individual's current health status, her risk of developing more serious disease associated with prolonged low levels of estrogen, and the possibility that potential benefits of treatment outweigh the risks for her. If estrogen is not an option, there are many other effective options. A woman's decision about hormone therapy may also change as more is learned through clinical trials and/or as personal situations and risk factors change.

Progestogen & HRT

Treatment that combines ERT plus a progestogen is called hormone replacement therapy or HRT. When a woman with a uterus chooses to use ERT, the progesterone that the ovaries once produced must be replaced to help counteract the increased risk of uterine cancer from taking ERT alone. Replacement therapy is available as progesterone or as progestin (synthetic progesterone). Both forms are called progestogens. Women who have had their uterus removed (hysterectomy) are not at risk for uterine cancer and, thus, have no reason to take progestogen with ERT.

Estrogen was prescribed alone (without a progestogen) in the United States until the early 1970s, when the associated increase in uterine cancer was recognized. Researchers found that combining a progestogen with ERT kept the endometrium from thickening, which essentially eliminated the risk of uterine cancer from ERT use. FDA-approved progestins (synthetic progestogens) were used initially because they were the only kind of progestogen that could be taken orally. More recently, micronized progesterone has become available in an FDA-approved oral formulation. Today, there are several progestogen options to allow tailoring to a woman's unique needs.

Uterine bleeding. In most women, using a progestogen causes the endometrium to shed and pass from the uterus as bleeding, similar to a menstrual period, although fertility is not restored. Some women find this progestogen-induced bleeding unacceptable, although the bleeding often decreases or stops over time. For many women, it is difficult to decide whether to tolerate the bleeding in exchange for estrogen's benefits, including relief from hot flashes and prevention of future diseases, such as osteoporosis.

Newer dosage schedules that combine estrogen and progestogen daily can eventually result in no uterine bleeding in some women while still protecting the lining of the uterus from becoming cancerous. However, many women, particularly those recently menopausal, do have vaginal spotting and bleeding during the first six months of the regimen. Each woman will develop her own typical bleeding pattern

when taking HRT. Any change from that pattern should be reported to her clinician right away.

There are various HRT schedules that can be used. Each woman should feel comfortable exploring different options with her clinician to determine which is best for her. These schedules include the following:

- **Cyclic HRT** provides estrogen for 25 days each month, adding progestogen on the last 10 to 14 days, followed by three to six days of no therapy. Thus, both hormones are "cycled." The popularity of this regimen has waned because of uterine bleeding each month when the progestogen cycle ends and the possibility of hot flashes returning during the therapy-free interval.

- **Continuous-cyclic HRT** (sometimes called sequential HRT) provides estrogen every day, with progestogen added for 10 to 14 days each month. With this regimen, uterine bleeding occurs in about 80% of women when the progestogen cycle ends each month.

- **Continuous-combined HRT** provides both hormones every day. The daily dose of progestogen

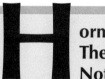

Hormone Replacement Therapy (HRT) Is Not A Contraceptive

Estrogens and progestogens are used in HRT to treat menopause-related changes; these hormones are also in most birth control pills. However, the doses of estrogen and progestogen used as HRT are not high enough to provide birth control. The doses used in birth control pills are about four or five times higher. Until menopause is reached (12 straight months without periods), hormonal or nonhormonal contraception must be used to avoid an unwanted pregnancy (see Birth Control As Menopause Approaches).

used is much lower than the daily doses used in cyclic therapy, resulting in a lower cumulative dose over a month's time. Progestogen can stimulate bleeding, but since it is taken every day, the timing of uterine bleeding is unpredictable. With this regimen, bleeding occurs in about 50% of women, perhaps more in recently postmenopausal women. After several months of therapy, uterine bleeding often stops. However, the uterus is still protected from estrogen's effect on cancer risk. US women have been choosing this regimen more and more.

• **Intermittent-combined HRT** is a new regimen (available as Ortho-Prefest) that provides estrogen every day, then adds progestogen intermittently in cycles of three days on, three days off. The cumulative monthly dose of progestogen is half that of a daily, continuous pattern. Bleeding and endometrial protection are similar to that with a continuous-combined regimen. Some studies suggest that this regimen is better at preserving the beneficial effects of estrogen on cholesterol, thus helping heart health.

Dosage forms of progestogen and HRT.
Progestogen is available in different forms – either alone or in combination with estrogen – allowing for individualized therapy (see charts). Not all progestogens are good choices for endometrial protection, but they can be used for other indications.

Progestogens are also available in custom-made formulations prepared by a compounding pharmacist following a healthcare provider's prescription.

Progestogen Products Commonly Used In The United States

PROGESTOGEN TYPE	PRODUCT NAME
Progestin: Oral Tablet	
medroxyprogesterone acetate	Amen, Cycrin, Provera
norethindrone	Micronor, Nor-QD
norethindrone acetate	Aygestin
norgestrel	Ovrette
levonorgestrel	Norplant
megestrol acetate	Megace (not for uterine protection)
Progestin: Injectable	
medroxyprogesterone acetate	Depo-Provera (not for uterine protection)
Progestin: IUD	
levonorgestrel	Mirena
Progesterone: Oral Capsule	
progesterone USP (in peanut oil)	Prometrium
Progesterone: Vaginal Gel	
progesterone	Crinone
Progesterone: IUD	
progesterone	Progestasert

48

Progesterone creams that can be purchased over-the-counter may or may not contain progesterone. Even if they do, the amount of progesterone absorbed through the skin may not be sufficient to protect the uterus against cancer if estrogen is used.

Side effects. In addition to uterine bleeding, the following side effects, some of which are similar to those of the premenstrual syndrome (PMS), may be experienced with progestogen use:

• Fluid retention;

• Headache;

• Breast tenderness;

• Alterations in mood.

In some women, these side effects may be substantially reduced with the use of a natural progesterone instead of a synthetic progestin. In addition, unlike progestin, progesterone does not appear to lower HDL, the good cholesterol that increases when estrogen is taken alone. More research is needed to clarify the effects of these hormones on heart disease risk.

Using progestogen is a complicated issue that depends, in part, on the type and dose of estrogen being used. The contraindications for treatment with progestogen are generally the same as those for estrogen.

Dealing with ERT/HRT Side Effects

There are various strategies to deal with the side effects that may occur with the use of ERT or HRT (see box on page 50). Many side effects are

Estrogen Plus Progestogen (HRT) Products FDA-Approved For Postmenopausal Use

REGIMEN	COMPOSITION	PRODUCT NAME
Oral: Continuous-Cyclic	conjugated equine estrogens and medroxyprogesterone acetate	Premphase
Oral: Continuous-Combined	conjugated equine estrogens and medroxyprogesterone acetate	Prempro
	ethinyl estradiol and norethindrone acetate	Femhrt
	17-beta-estradiol and norethindrone acetate	Activella
Oral: Intermittent-Combined	17-beta-estradiol and norgestimate	Ortho-Prefest
Skin Patch: Continuous-Cyclic	17-beta-estradiol and norethindrone acetate	CombiPatch
Skin Patch: Continuous-Combined	17-beta-estradiol and norethindrone acetate	CombiPatch

temporary until a woman adjusts to the hormonal changes. Unless side effects are severe, a trial of three months of hormonal therapy is advised to see if side effects resolve. One strategy is appropriate for any side effect: stop ERT/HRT (by tapering slowly) to see if hormones are the cause, because side effects could be the result of something else.

Androgen

Many women are surprised to learn that androgen, which is considered primarily a male hormone, is also a female hormone. It is secreted by the ovaries as testosterone and androstenedione. Aging ovaries produce less androgen as well as less estrogen, although the decline is not so steep as with estrogen. Conditions that accelerate the decline of internal androgen levels include surgical removal of one or both ovaries prior to menopause, pituitary

and adrenal insufficiency, corticosteroid therapy, and some chronic illnesses. Because of the lack of androgen, some women suffer a decline in sex drive. Androgen therapy may help. Some women have also reported an increase in energy while taking androgen. However, androgen therapy is appropriate only when a woman is also using estrogen – never androgen alone.

There have been many studies in which androgen was added to estrogen therapy for menopausal women. Currently, the only androgen-containing product that is FDA-approved for use in women is Estratest, a prescription oral tablet containing an androgen (methyltestosterone) and an estrogen (esterified estrogens). However, no product, including Estratest, is FDA-approved for boosting sex drive in women. Estratest is approved for the treatment of hot flashes that are unresponsive to

Side Effects Strategies With ERT/HRT Therapy

Fluid retention. Restrict salt intake, maintain adequate water intake, exercise, try a mild diuretic.

Bloating. Lower the estrogen dose, switch to another estrogen, switch from oral estrogen to a skin patch, lower the progestogen dose, switch to progesterone or another progestin.

Breast tenderness. Restrict salt intake, cut down on caffeine and chocolate, lower the estrogen dose, switch to another estrogen, switch from oral estrogen to a skin patch, switch to progesterone or another progestin.

Headaches. Restrict salt, caffeine, and alcohol intake, ensure adequate water intake, lower the dose of estrogen and/or progestogen, switch to a continuous dosage schedule or a skin patch to avoid hormone fluctuations.

Mood changes. Restrict salt, caffeine, and alcohol intake, ensure adequate water intake, lower the progestogen dose, switch to progesterone, switch to a continuous dosage schedule or to a skin patch to avoid hormone fluctuations, exercise regularly.

Nausea. Take oral estrogen tablets with meals, lower the estrogen and/or progestogen dose, switch to another estrogen, switch from oral estrogen to a skin patch.

Skin irritation under patch. Switch to a patch with a different adhesive, apply patch to a different area, change to oral estrogen.

ERT alone. Some women, however, find that sex drive is improved by taking this product.

A skin patch product containing another androgen (testosterone) is being developed. Testosterone products also can be custom-made by a compounding pharmacist following a healthcare provider's prescription. One popular form contains 1% to 2% micronized testosterone USP in a water-soluble base; this topical product can be absorbed by rubbing it on the skin. Other custom forms of testosterone include tablets, injections, or pellets implanted under the skin. As with all custom formulations that are not FDA-approved, therapy should be used with caution.

Dosage is very important. Too much androgen may not provide the desired improvement in sex drive and can cause feelings of agitation, aggression, and/or depression. Higher dosages can also cause facial and body hair growth, acne, an enlarged clitoris, a lowered voice, and muscle weight gain. These side effects may not go away after therapy stops. Androgen may adversely affect some of estrogen's heart health benefits, even more so than progestin. Caution is recommended when considering this type of hormone treatment because the safety of taking androgen for extended periods of time has not been established.

Women must not use the androgen products FDA-approved for men, as these contain very high doses that would be harmful to women. However, several new products are being studied for use in women, and will, hopefully, be on the market in the near future.

Other Prescription Therapies

Treatments for menopause can be aimed at menopause disturbances or targeted to prevent the potential long-term effects of lowered estrogen levels. An array of remedies is available today, and more are under study for future use.

Although not FDA-approved for this use, low-dose oral contraceptives containing estrogen and progestin are prescribed to help regulate periods, reduce hot flashes, improve sleep, and level out mood swings. Oral contraceptives, even those with very low hormone doses, provide significantly more hormone than standard HRT regimens. Since the lowest effective dose of any drug should always be used to reduce exposure to risk, women who need to continue with HRT are switched from oral contraceptives to HRT after menopause is reached. However, a woman taking birth control pills will continue to have uterine bleeding even after menopause, making it difficult to determine that menopause has occurred. Thus, many clinicians make the switch automatically at age 51 – the average age of menopause.

Several other prescription drugs are available as options to ERT/HRT in treating hot flashes, but they are not FDA-approved for this use (see Hot Flashes).

COMPLEMENTARY & ALTERNATIVE MEDICINES

Therapies considered by some to differ from traditional medical treatments are referred to as complementary and alternative medicine (CAM) therapies. These nonprescription treatments are promoted for a range of menopause symptoms, and the remedy usually depends on the specific complaint. The effect, if any, of CAM therapies may take several weeks. In contrast, prescription hormones usually begin to take effect within a few days. Some CAM therapies are expensive and many are untested. CAM therapies include foods, herbs and other botanicals (plant sources), and supplements. Often, a pharmacist or herbalist can offer advice on their use. CAM therapies can also include naturopathy, homeopathy, and acupuncture, each practiced by specialists in the field.

Many CAM therapies are advertised as "natural." This marketing word is used because many consumers believe it suggests that a product that's natural is better or safer. However, this may not be the case. CAM therapies may actually be more dangerous than prescription drugs because less is known about them, and their purity, dosage, and advertising claims are not regulated by the FDA.

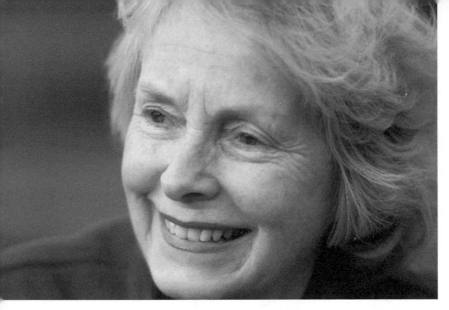

These products are marketed as dietary supplements (see Nonprescription Therapies). Women need to use the same caution with CAM therapies as with all other therapies.

As more research findings accumulate to support their effectiveness, some therapies now listed as CAM therapies will undoubtedly be moved from the CAM category to mainstream. Some CAM therapies may be proven to be ineffective or too risky, and they will not be included anywhere in a listing of menopause treatment options. Still others will remain classified as CAM, since not all therapies can be adequately tested, often because of lack of financial backing for studies since many CAM products are not patent-protected and, thus, do not allow marketers to recoup their research investment.

Phytoestrogens & Soy

Currently, intensive research is focused on phytoestrogens (plant estrogens), such as isoflavones. These are naturally occurring compounds found in rich supply in soybeans, soy products, and red clover. They are similar in chemical structure to estrogen and can produce weak estrogen-like effects. There is some evidence that eating soy foods (such as tofu, tempeh, soy milk, or roasted soy nuts) may be helpful in reducing hot flashes and other menopause effects. The most convincing beneficial health effects have been attributed to the actions of soy foods on fats in the blood, stimulating the FDA to recommend eating a daily serving of soy foods (25 grams of "soy protein"), as part of a diet low in saturated fat and cholesterol, to help lower the risk of heart disease. There are inadequate data to evaluate the effect of soy/isoflavones on vaginal dryness, bone mass, and breast cancer.

Commercial preparations containing isoflavones — including over-the-counter supplements, additives to "multi" supplements, and fortified foods (such as candy bars) — are marketed to provide similar health benefits. It is not clear, however, whether the observed health benefits sometimes seen with soy foods are caused from the isoflavones alone or from isoflavones plus other components in whole foods. Until the effectiveness and long-term safety of isoflavone supplements have been clearly established, eating reasonable amounts of soy food is probably a better choice. Foods have widely different amounts of isoflavone (see box), and there is great variability within the same food type, depending on many factors, such as growing conditions.

Botanicals

A number of botanical (plant-based) products, including herbs and multi-herb products, have been used to treat acute menopause-related conditions, such as hot flashes. They are not meant to be considered for prevention of serious diseases, such as osteoporosis. There is limited research information documenting effectiveness and safety of these products. All are regulated as dietary supplements, not as drugs. None are regulated for purity, dose, or health claims.

The most widely used products include the following:

Black cohosh (*Cimicifuga racemosa*), also known as black snakeroot and bugbane, is available in several forms. The most studied form is an extract used in Germany. The typical dose is 160 mg/day. The most well-known brand is Remifemin. **Pros:** There are reports of effectiveness with hot flashes, vaginal dryness, and depression, and some clinical studies support these reports, although critics contend the studies are poorly designed. Results are evident within two to four weeks. Side effects are rare and include gastrointestinal upset, typically with first-time use. **Cons:** Black cohosh should not be used longer than six months. It should not be used in combination with ERT/HRT or with antihypertensive medications.

Isoflavone Content Of Food

Food	Average Isoflavone Amount (mg) in Food (100 g)
Soybeans, green, raw	151.17
Soy flour	148.61
Soy protein isolate	97.43
Miso soup	60.39
Tempeh	43.52
Soybeans, sprouted, raw	40.71
Tofu, silken	27.91
Tofu yogurt	16.30
Soy hot dog	15.00
Soy milk	9.65
Soy sauce, shoyu	1.64

Dong quai (*Angelica sinensis*), also known as Chinese angelica, tang-kuei, and dang-gui, is used for menstrual cycle regulation, easing cramps, and menopausal symptoms. **Pros:** Some women report effectiveness for these conditions. **Cons:** One study using 4.5 grams/day for 12 weeks found it to be no more effective than placebo in relieving hot flashes. Dong quai, however, is not meant to be used alone but in an individually tailored herb mixture.

Evening primrose oil (*Oenethera biennis*) comes from seeds rich in linoleic acid. It is used at 1,500-3,000 mg/day for relief of hot flashes. **Pros:** Some women report effectiveness. **Cons:** There is no scientific evidence that effectiveness is better than placebo. Side effects include inflammation, nausea, diarrhea, blood clots, and lowered immune system. Women with epilepsy or those using phenothiazines or blood thinners (including aspirin and warfarin as well as supplements of vitamin E, feverfew, garlic, or ginger) should not use this product.

Ginkgo (*Ginkgo biloba*) is an antioxidant used for short-term memory loss. **Pros:** Some studies document effectiveness. **Cons:** Bleeding is a serious side effect. Women using blood thinners should not use this product. Use must be discontinued for two to three weeks before and after surgery. Use is not recommended for menopause symptoms.

Ginseng (*Panax ginseng*) is a term used to describe many different herbs used for preventing age-related cognitive decline, fatigue, and building resistance to viruses. **Pros:** Some women report effectiveness. **Cons:** There is a lack of scientific evidence to support these claims. Side effects include vaginal bleeding, worsening of menopause symptoms, high blood pressure, headache, aggressive behavior, mental disturbances, and insomnia. Ginseng should not be used with stimulants, diabetic agents, phenelzine

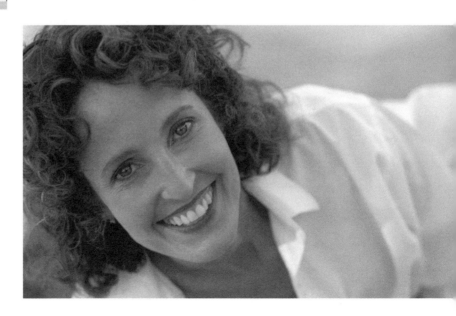

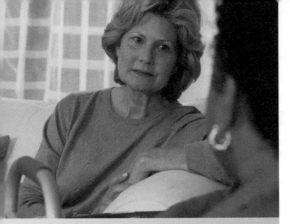

(a potent antidepressant), blood thinners, or diuretics. Use is not recommended because of side effects and lack of efficacy data.

Kava (*Piper methysticum*), sometimes called kava kava, is used for menstrual cramps, muscle tension, and insomnia. **Pros:** Studies with postmenopausal women document efficacy in relieving mild anxiety. **Cons:** Kava may be addictive and must be used with caution. Mild gastrointestinal upset has been reported; long-term use can cause yellow, scaly skin. Kava should not be used with any medication taken for psychological problems, antihistamines, or alcohol.

St. John's wort (*Hypericum perforatum*) is used for mild to moderate depression at a dose of 300 mg taken three times daily. **Pros:** Studies show effectiveness. **Cons:** Side effects include gastrointestinal upset, fatigue, and increased sensitivity to sunlight. When taking this herb, sunblock, a hat, and wraparound sunglasses should be worn when in the sun and sunbathing must be avoided. St. John's wort should not be used with drugs for psychological problems or HIV, or after organ transplant.

Wild yam (*Dioscorea villosa*) must be processed chemically in a lab to the hormone progesterone; humans lack the chemicals necessary to make this change. Some products are marketed with claims of relieving hot flashes, among others. **Pros:** None. **Cons:** There is no scientific evidence that wild yam is effective.

DIFFERENT WOMEN, DIFFERENT NEEDS

For most women experiencing natural menopause, the decision to seek treatment is based on the severity of short-term complaints, risk of disease in later years, and personal attitudes about menopause and medication. Regardless of the severity of health complaints, women in perimenopause should consult a healthcare provider.

Some women in perimenopause find adequate help from nonprescription remedies, such as vitamins and herbs. Others choose prescription hormones, either ERT/HRT or oral contraceptives, during this transition. Following perimenopause, some women choose ERT/HRT or more targeted prescription therapies to protect against osteoporosis and, possibly, heart disease.

Prescription ERT/HRT appears to be the treatment of choice for women who experience premature menopause (either natural or induced) because of their increased risk for osteoporosis and heart disease.

However, it is also important to assess and improve overall diet, exercise regimen, and other lifestyle factors. For all women, living a healthy lifestyle can contribute significantly to improved well-being, not only today but throughout life.

COMMITTING TO TREATMENT

Prior to beginning any treatment or combination of treatments, whether intended to alleviate short-term disturbances or prevent diseases later in life, a woman needs to be assured that the treatment regimen selected is the best for her. This requires an open discussion with her healthcare provider about her health status and concerns and in-depth information on available treatment options. A clinician with expertise in managing menopause can offer optimal care.

It Takes Time

For optimal results, treatment takes time. It takes time for effects to manifest fully and for side effects to diminish. For example, the effects of ERT/HRT usually become stable after six to eight weeks.

Nonprescription and CAM therapies, on the other hand, may take months for the desired effects, if any.

Over time, therapy may need to change because of gradually lowering levels of ovarian hormones and the possible appearance of medical conditions unrelated to menopause or menopause treatments. Also, new research and changing ideas about medicines and health arise that have an impact on health decisions.

Before switching from one therapy to another, a "wash-out" period during which no drugs are used may be required to clear all drugs from the body. If ERT/HRT is to be discontinued, it should be tapered off in order to avoid severe recurrence of hot flashes.

Treatment should last as long as it is needed. Duration will be different for each woman, depending on her own unique and ongoing health profile, and risks of developing serious diseases later in life. Because of this, regular checkups are important throughout life.

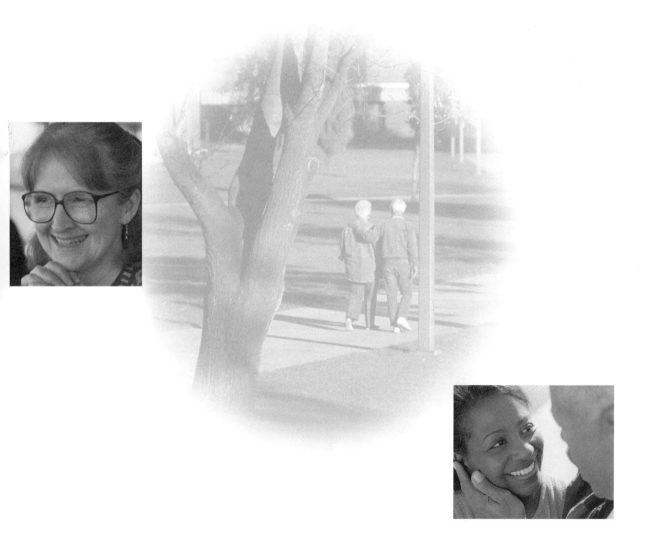

ACHIEVING OPTIMAL HEALTH

EACH WOMAN'S MENOPAUSE

EXPERIENCE IS DIFFERENT. THE GREATEST

DIFFERENCES OBSERVED ARE BETWEEN

WOMEN WHO HAVE NATURAL

MENOPAUSE AT THE TYPICAL TIME

AND THOSE WHOSE MENOPAUSE IS

EARLY OR INDUCED.

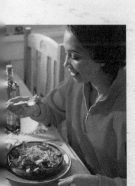

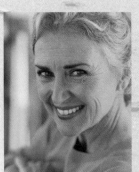

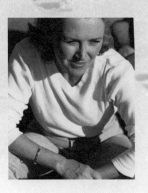

Many women go through natural menopause with minimal discomfort during the perimenopausal years. For most, the disturbances diminish or disappear over time, or they are reduced with lifestyle changes, such as exercise and diet modification. With treatment, most disturbances decrease or disappear. Some women need treatment and should not feel as if they have "failed" to manage menopause on their own. Their unique makeup makes them different, and unique treatment is required.

There is no single way to ensure the best possible quality of life through perimenopause and beyond. Not only is each woman unique, but therapeutic options keep changing. Research will continue to provide better guidelines, so women can work along with their healthcare providers to determine their individual health status and their risk factors for developing diseases in the years to come. It is beneficial for a woman to invest time working with a healthcare professional who is willing to listen, to help determine special needs, and to recommend therapeutic adjustments that are required as a woman's body continues to change in its own individual way.

KEYS TO HEALTH

Healthy behaviors and regular clinical exams are the keys to health. Women of all ages, whether perimenopausal or postmenopausal, require an annual physical exam by a healthcare provider. During this checkup, the clinician will need information on:

• Health history, personal and family;

• Health concerns or current problems;

• Diet;

• Level of physical activity;

• Smoking status;

• Drugs and health remedies being used;

• All healthcare practitioners currently being consulted.

During the checkup, various tests can be performed to determine heart, bone, breast, pelvic, and rectal health. Pap tests are important even after menopause because they screen for precancerous conditions of the cervix. Annual mammograms are important for women aged 40 and over. Height measurements are needed since loss of height may be indicative of osteoporosis. Blood, urine, and other lab tests may be needed to uncover certain diseases or risks of diseases, such as diabetes, thyroid disease, urogenital infection, colorectal cancer, and heart disease. Hormone level measurements may be helpful, but they can be misleading because hormone levels can fluctuate and testing can be unreliable.

During the checkup, immunizations to prevent infectious diseases can be updated, and various key health components can be discussed, such as:

• Sexuality;

• Exercise;

• Alcohol use or abuse;

• Drug use or abuse;

• Physical abuse;

• Reducing stress;

• Improving sleep;

• Smoking cessation;

• Attaining ideal weight;

• Maintaining ideal weight;

• Obtaining adequate nutrition;

• Obtaining sufficient calcium.

There is no average woman. Each woman is unique and requires attention to her special needs.

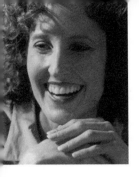

During the checkup, various treatment options can also be presented, if needed. Treatment plans should include the following:

- Discussion of risks and benefits;

- A plan to watch for side effects;

- A plan to monitor outcomes;

- Possible alternatives.

A TIME OF NEW BEGINNINGS

Perimenopause is an ideal time to begin or to reinforce a health promotion program that will serve a woman throughout the remainder of life. Most postmenopausal women view menopause as the beginning of many positive changes in their lives and health. In this youth-valued society, a woman's perception of menopause can be influenced by many negative stereotypes proliferated by peer groups, family, media, and health professionals. But education and counseling can dispel myths and challenge outdated stereotypes.

A recent NAMS survey found that US midlife women were divided in their views of menopause. Some consider it a medical condition requiring treatment, while others view it as a natural transition that should be managed by natural means. One recent mail survey found that

Menopause can mark the beginning of an exciting new time of life.

women want more information about menopause, but their major source of information has been consumer magazines, not their healthcare providers. This survey also found that women have serious misunderstandings about their health risks after menopause.

It's also important to realize the vast diversity in women and how social and cultural differences between and among groups of women could have an impact not only on the way women experience menopause and view treatments, but also on their future health and well-being. Risk factors, patterns of disease and mortality, access to health care, economic status, therapies, and norms related to femininity and aging all differ among these groups. There is very little research, however, on how these differences relate to menopause. By far, menopause research has focused on Caucasian, middle-class women. Although more diverse populations are now being studied, considerable information is needed before every woman can be optimally helped.

As women experience the physical, emotional, and social changes of approaching menopause, they face a unique opportunity to identify their own strategies for midlife wellness. Each woman is the expert on her own body — and, as this expert, she will benefit more if she's well informed. The primary message for women at this stage of life is that they can enjoy their bodies well into old age, provided they make informed, responsible choices.

ADDITIONAL RESOURCES

WOMEN'S HEALTH

The North American Menopause Society (NAMS)
P.O. Box 94527
Cleveland, OH 44101
440-442-7550
800-774-5342 (toll-free automated consumer line)
www.menopause.org
Most comprehensive selection of menopause information, including referral and suggested reading lists.

**American College of Obstetricians
& Gynecologists Resource Center (ACOG)**
P.O. Box 96920
Washington, DC 20090
www.acog.org

**American Society for Reproductive Medicine
(ASRM)**
1209 Montgomery Highway
Birmingham, AL 35216
205-978-5000
www.asrm.org

**Association of Reproductive Health Professionals
(ARHP)**
2401 Pennsylvania Avenue, NW, Suite 350
Washington, DC 20037
202-466-3825
800-804-7374 (toll-free)
www.arhp.org

**Association of Women's Health,
Obstetric & Neonatal Nurses (AWHONN)**
2000 L Street, NW, Suite 740
Washington, DC 20036
202-261-2400
800-673-8499 (toll-free)

The Hormone Foundation
4350 East West Highway, Suite 500
Bethesda, MD 20814
800-HORMONE (toll-free)
www.hormone.org

The Jacobs Institute of Women's Health
409 12th Street, SW
Washington, DC 20024
202-863-4990

**National Association for Women's Health
(NAWH)**
300 West Adams, Suite 328
Chicago, IL 60606
312-786-1468
www.nawh.org

**National Association of Nurse Practitioners
in Women's Health**
503 Capitol Court, NE, Suite 300
Washington, DC 20002
202-543-9693
www.npwh.org

National Women's Health Network
514 10th Street, NW, Suite 400
Washington, DC 20004
202-628-7814 (Tues/Thurs only)
www.womenshealthnetwork.org

National Women's Health Resource Center
120 Albany Street, Suite 820
New Brunswick, NJ 08901
877-986-9472 (toll-free)
www.healthywomen.org

Planned Parenthood Federation of America
800-230-PLAN (toll-free) for medical questions, local clinics, and information.
www.plannedparenthood.org

**The Society of Obstetricians and
Gynecologists of Canada (SOGC)**
780 Echo Drive
Ottawa, ON K1S 5N8
613-730-4192
800-561-2416 (toll-free, Canada only)
www.sogc.org

CANCER

American Cancer Society
800-ACS-2345 (toll-free)
www.cancer.org

Canadian Breast Cancer Foundation
790 Bay Street, Suite 1000
Toronto, ON M5G 1N8
800-387-9816 (toll-free, Canada only)
www.cbcf.org

Canadian Cancer Society
10 Alcorn Avenue, Suite 200
Toronto, ON M4V 3B1
416-961-7223
888-939-3333 (toll-free, Canada only)
www.cancer.ca

Cancer Information Service
National Cancer Institute
800-4-CANCER (toll-free)
www.nci.nih.gov

Gynecologic Cancer Foundation
401 North Michigan Avenue
Chicago, IL 60611
800-444-4441 (toll-free)
www.wcn.org/gcf

HEART DISEASE

American Heart Association
7272 Greenville Avenue
Dallas, TX 75231
214-373-6300
800-AHA-USA1 (toll-free)
www.americanheart.org

The Heart and Stroke Foundation of Canada
222 Queen Street, Suite 1402
Ottawa, ON KIP 5V9
613-569-4361
888-473-4636 (toll-free, Canada only)
www.heartandstroke.ca

National Heart, Lung, and Blood Institute
P.O. Box 30105
Bethesda, MD 20824
301-592-8573
www.nhlbi.nih.gov

SLEEP

National Sleep Foundation
1522 K Street, NW, Suite 500
Washington, DC 20005
www.sleepfoundation.org

STOPPING SMOKING

American Lung Association
1740 Broadway
New York, NY 10019
212-315-8700
800-LUNG-USA (toll-free)
www.lungusa.org

MENTAL HEALTH

American Psychiatric Association
1400 K Street, NW
Washington, DC 20005
202-682-6000
888-357-PSYCH (toll-free)
www.psych.org

American Psychological Association
750 First Street, NE
Washington, DC 20002
800-964-2000 (toll-free)
www.apa.org

Canadian Mental Health Association
2160 Yonge Street, 3rd Floor
Toronto, ON M4S 2Z3
416-484-7750
www.cmha.ca

National Institute of Mental Health
NIMH Public Inquiries
6001 Executive Boulevard
Room 8184, MSC 9663
Bethesda, MD 20892
301-443-4513
www.nimh.nih.gov

OSTEOPOROSIS

National Osteoporosis Foundation (NOF)
1232 22nd Street, NW
Washington, DC 20037
202-223-2226
www.nof.org

Osteoporosis Society of Canada
33 Laird Drive
Toronto, ON M4G 3S9
416-696-2663
800-977-1778 (toll-free, Canada only, French)
800-463-6842 (toll-free, Canada only, English)
www.osteoporosis.ca

SEX ISSUES

**Sexuality Information & Education
Council of the U.S. (SIECUS)**
130 West 42nd Street, Suite 350
New York, NY 10036
212-819-9770
www.siecus.org

UROGENITAL HEALTH

Interstitial Cystitis Association
51 Monroe Street, Suite 1402
Rockville, MD 20850
301-610-5300
800-HELP-ICA (toll-free)
www.ichelp.com

National Association for Continence
P.O. Box 8306
Spartanburg, SC 29305
800-BLADDER (toll-free)
www.nafc.org

National Vulvodynia Association
P.O. Box 4491
Silver Spring, MD 20914
301-299-0775
www.nva.org

The Simon Foundation for Continence
P.O. Box 835
Wilmette, IL 60091
800-23-SIMON (toll-free)
www.simonfoundation.org

The Vulvar Pain Foundation
P.O. Box 177
Graham, NC 27253
336-226-0704
www.vulvarpainfoundation.org